WHAT IS GLUTEN AND WHAT IS GLUTEN IN

BY JAQUI KARR, C.S.N., C.V.D.

The human body is engineered to be healthy and happy.

...and then human engineering gets in the way...

JAQUI KARR

http://JaquiKarr.com

CONTENTS

HOW I ALMOST DIED FROM GLUTEN

"You're not 20 anymore."

...that was the brilliant diagnosis of the first medical doctor I went to when I went from being a healthy athletic individual to suddenly experiencing migraines, constant pain, cramps, bloating, and other symptoms I'd rather not mention. Not 20 anymore... apparently incessant pain was normal at the very old age of 38.

Had healthy-to-sick been a gradual transition over years, I might have hesitated to listen to him for a few seconds, but it was literally overnight. I remember clear as day the exact moment it all began.

It was August 2008 and I was looking forward to my usual mountain run after work. But there was a torrential downpour of rain that evening so I decided to work out at the gym instead. In the middle of my workout I suddenly experienced a pain I had never felt before. The best way to describe it is what it must feel like to be hit in the back of the head by a baseball bat - not exactly a typical headache. At first I thought someone in the gym was walking around with a body bar and accidentally actually hit me. I looked behind me but no one was there.

The pain was sharp, immobilizing, and lasted about 15 minutes. I sat on a bench waiting for it to go away not even trusting myself to walk down to the locker room.

That sharp blunt pain turned into a migraine that lasted days but I didn't give it much thought until other symptoms started popping up one by one. The migraine became an incessant relentless headache. Then came stomach cramps, bloating, and the return of eczema (which I hadn't seen since childhood).

Within weeks of that initial sharp pain to the back of my head I knew something was very wrong and went to see a doctor. He took a blood test, said I was the healthiest person he ever saw and these little things were normal as we age. Normal? Little things?

The second and third doctors echoed each other with the same thing, "Well you're not getting any younger". ?!? *Happy Birthday to me.* But as the days went on, things got much worse.

By October of that same year I was in so much pain I found myself canceling business trips, not working the long hours I was used to, not exercising at all, and spending a lot of time in bed. I also noticed I was losing weight inexplicably. My eating habits hadn't changed very much but I had completely stopped exercising - simple math says I should have been gaining, not losing weight.

This might be a good time to stop and mention that I had never experienced sickness of any kind before. My friends used to call me "Iron Woman"; I was strong and athletic my entire life. The worst thing that would happen about once a decade was I would get a little cold, sneeze for a few days, and it would be over. So to go from incredibly healthy to *this,* overnight, was quite surreal. And boy was I ever inexperienced with doctors.

By the end of October I was 15 pounds lighter, in constant pain, and now experiencing dizzy spells which soon led to fainting, which led me to the emergency room of a hospital. The months that followed were mind boggling to me.

On that first hospital visit they ran a cat-scan, told me everything was normal, and sent me home with instructions to see my family doctor (which I didn't have since I was never sick). The doctors I had seen were just friend's recommendations and one came out of the phone book. None had any answers. I didn't know where to turn but things rapidly got worse still.

Now November, and the dizzy spells came more often and another fainting episode landed me back in the hospital. This time the doctor spent more than 2 minutes with me and when I told him about the weight loss (20+lbs at that point) he decided to test for cancer and I was sent home once again. Weeks later, the results were negative. But my decline continued.

Within a few weeks I was unable to work full days anymore and now became very scared with more and more symptoms appearing week after week. The left side of my body started going numb, I mean I couldn't feel my own hand as I washed my face numb. Zero feeling – it's scary. My leg and arm had been feeling tingly but when I discovered my face had no sense of feeling at all, it was back to the E.R. They ran an EKG and eliminated the possibility of a stroke.

The E.R. doctor said tingling and numbness were congruent with Multiple Sclerosis (goodness forbid we connect the dots and think of a nutritional deficiency). While MS does cause tingling and numbness, so does a vitamin B_{12} deficiency. Since I had several "normal" blood test results just within 60 days, we weren't doing any more blood work, so deficiencies fell off the radar.

You may be wondering why I didn't self diagnose. Well, three reasons:

1) The fact that it all started with a migraine and was mainly a head issue in the beginning threw me off track – I thought it was neurological

2) It never occurred to me so much havoc could be created from a food issue – and my diet hadn't changed at all, so why would I suspect food?

3) I had never heard of Celiac or its symptoms

An MRI confirmed I did not have MS. Fantastic. It's not MS. But what is it? Half a dozen doctors are telling me everything is normal and yet my life is dispersing in front of my very eyes, the left part of my body is going numb, and if I lose any more weight I know that I will be staring at organ failure.

Where do I turn to? Emergency rooms can't help as they are drastically overcrowded and their sole job is to make sure you are breathing so they can get to the bleeding head trauma patient. If you can stand upright, you're sent home. GP's are hard to come by and several have already poked and prodded to tell me I am fine – yet clearly...

I must mention that every GP I saw were ready to prescribe pain killers and when I asked them if we could find the root cause instead of masking it, they just shrugged and said "see a specialist". But my symptoms being head to toe, we had no idea what was wrong so they couldn't refer me to a specialist. What a circle.

Same for the E.R., they were happy to put morphine into the I.V. while rehydrating me but no one seemed interested in what was causing the pain or dehydration.

Had it not been for my healthy and organic lifelong habits which I adamantly refused to change, I would probably have been too drugged to be writing this right now and battling a whole new myriad of medical problems... *IF I was still alive at all*. I found it downright shocking how fast those prescription pads came out.

The fact is that with my knowledge of nutrition and fitness I should have been able to self-diagnose; what threw me off was the incredibly rapid decline and the extreme levels of pain. I sincerely thought something major had happened and I had contracted some terminal illness, all this havoc couldn't be coming from something as simple as food intolerance, right?

At the 5 month mark of doctors, clinics, emergency rooms, cat-scans, MRI's, blood tests, an EKG, ultrasounds, x-rays *(I should have been glowing in the dark at that point)* I found myself back at square one: agonizing pain and no answers.

Finally one cold windy December night I found myself sitting on the floor of my living room, just out of yet another E.R. visit, clinically depressed (another side effect of malnutrition and gut imbalance), crying uncontrollably and staring into my blurred fireplace. After what seems like hours, in that one broken down moment of despair I found clarity. I stopped expecting resolve from any outside source and asked myself what was wrong. And I knew. In an instant, I knew.

This wasn't neurological, it wasn't a horrible thing I had contracted, it was simply overall exhaustion and my body's immune system gave out. Something pushed my body to failure and although it could have reacted any one of hundreds of ways, it reacted by being unable to process food anymore. I thought it was *all* food at that point, I thought my entire digestive system was in failure mode.

I remembered something I once read: "your body is always in perfect health if you just stay out of its way."

Genetic disposition or not, our horrible food supply is definitely getting in the way of health. My love of pizza and fabulous artisan breads had caught up to me.

Through streaming tears I sat there in front of that fire and created a time line. I wrote down everything that happened in the order that it happened. Every symptom I felt, every unsubstantiated feeling I had.

I proceeded to book a triple session with a new private doctor. I remember the receptionist telling me initial consultations were usually 20 minutes and I gave her my credit card number over the phone and said "I need one full hour of the doctor's undivided attention, just charge me in advance whether we use the hour or not."

Three days later I sat in his office, told him I knew I had weakened my own immune system, told him I knew this was a digestive issue, told him the long list of problems it was not, showed him my tear stained papers documenting the timeline of events, and made him hear out the whole sordid story.

After silently listening to me for half an hour he calmly said "I think I know what's wrong." 24 hours later the tTG blood test his clinic had run on the spot at that initial visit pointed to gluten.

Celiac Disease was later confirmed via biopsy.

Knowing what I know about the disease now, my extreme and rapid reaction was indeed highly rare.

The reason this last doctor suspected Celiac was because he ignored the last few months of the whole messy affair and focused on the beginning. Before showing him my timeline the first thing I did was put my hands on my gut and said "it started here, the really excruciating pain all started here, I think the migraines were only symptoms." *Apparently he listened.*

I may have broken a world record in fastest physical decline due to gluten reaction, but I probably also broke a record for fastest and most complete recovery. Though I did have an upper edge with a lot of food knowledge and a whole lot of tricks I developed quickly enough, starting with my initial recovery strategy.

The biggest challenge was finding a truly accurate list of what was safe to eat and what was not, and when this seemed like an impossible task I created one. There were too many flaws in all the lists I kept finding. I went raw for an entire year while I dedicated myself to researching item by item; in the end I knew exactly what was safe or not, and you have it here in this book.

I returned to a healthy weight, I got my life back, I learned how to handle the social aspects of being a food outcast, I learned more than I ever wanted to know about illness – and I committed to helping others find fantastic health too. Whether their decline comes from an auto-immune disorder or just bad eating habits, anyone who wants to be well, can be.

As someone who knocked on death's door and came back to feel stronger than ever, the most important thing I have to say is if I can be well again, anyone can.

If I can go from an emaciated skeleton needing I.V.'s to stay hydrated to six months later kayaking intensely for three+ hours, *believe me*, you can feel like a million bucks too.

So as I reflect on my entire Dance With Celiac Disease from "you're not 20 anymore" to when I now hear "one little bite won't hurt you" *(if only they knew what that one little bite could trigger),* I have one thing left to say:

It may be a lifelong dance I am in, but my Celiac dance partner will never lead again.

WHAT IS GLUTEN

A protein. Gluten is a protein.

...and there is a good reason I am starting out with a one-word explanation, I want it to be extra easy to understand, which we'll get to in a minute...

When people talk about avoiding gluten due to sensitivities or reactions, they are always focused on: 1) "gliadin" the protein found in wheat 2) "hordein" the protein found in barley 3) "secalin" the protein in rye.

So up to now the spotlight has been on wheat, barley, and rye. Avoid three things, simple, right? *Not so fast.*

Just those three alone get complicated when it comes to processed foods because so many ingredients are derivatives of them, particularly wheat and barley. Literally hundreds of commonly used by-products are found in thousands of every day (processed) foods. The "hidden sources" and "a to z list" sections of this book will show you how to stay 100% gluten free.

Let's get back to the protein issue and take a closer look at ALL grains. Going back several years, many studies have found all grains to cause issues similar to those of wheat, barley, and rye – and I'll quote them in the next chapter.

ALL GRAINS

I'll start with the bad news: the medical community has not conclusively taken a position on whether or not all grains are harmful, though many noted doctors seem to think they are (as of 2012, I doubt we'll see any such unanimous conclusion in the next decade or two).

This means the burden lies on you to decide. And this is why I began by saying "gluten is a protein"... a quick explanation so you can make an informed decision:

Several grains like corn and rice are generally "accepted" as safe yet all grains have gluten. The reason some have been labeled as safe is due to the lower levels of gluten or lower levels of glutamine.

"Prolamins" are: proteins high in **PROL**ine and glut**AMIN**e. Gliadin and glutenin are the prolamins for wheat, and this being the highest percentage of gluten within grains has become the focus of most studies, but gliadin is not the only offender to those who suffer from gluten issues.

There are studies[5,6,7,8,9] going back 20 years that show some patients react to corn, rice, and all other grains, but we don't know why some react and others do not. Issues to consider:

1) The body's immediate reaction, or lack thereof, (even with those who react acutely with higher

levels of gluten) is not a good measuring stick – harmful antibodies might still be created whether the person feels symptoms or not

2) The damage from inflammation (reaction to gluten) can be outright fatal. We need to take the matter seriously and proceed with caution

HERE ARE THE PROTEIN CONTENTS OF GRAINS:

Barley: hordein 45-55%
Corn: zein 55%
Millet*: panicin 20-40%
Oats: avenin 16%
Rice: orzenin 5%
Rye: secalin 30-50%
Sorgum: kafirin 52%
Wheat: gliadin 69%

*Millet may be a controversy within a controversy – some studies claim it has zero gluten because its prolamin is not "glutelin-like", particularly in the finger and foxtail varieties. These are generally older studies and not considering Celiac or Gluten Sensitivity.

These are just proteins we know of! A doctor at the University of Maryland discovered "zonulin", a protein that also causes a reaction if you're gluten sensitive. There is still a lot to be discovered.

Many of us rely heavily on rice when we eliminate other glutens from our diet, so yet another restriction is not welcome news. I'm with you!

If you have been gluten free for more than 6 months and still not feeling quite back to 100%, even if it is not full blown symptoms, perhaps eliminating all grains for 1-3 months would be a good experiment. If you find yourself feeling completely fantastic after a while, then you will know if grains work with you or not.

Clearly there are variables that differ from one person to another so while one may tolerate these grains well, another may not. Those variables are far from being clear. Right now the focus is on methods of testing, looking for certain genes, etc.

They claim we don't know what the long term effects of continuous digestion of small amounts of gluten are. Really? We don't? In the largest study[1] ever done on the issue they found mortality rates were higher for those with Celiac Disease and another study[2] showed that even when supposedly on a gluten free diet for 9.7 years less than half the patients had normalized.

Could it be that what we are considering "gluten free" is actually not gluten free? And could the "legal" amounts of gluten be too high? I will cover the latter part in a later chapter called "the law".

Consider using quinoa, chia seeds, chick pea flour, bean flours, lentils... basically replace all grains with seeds and legumes if you truly want to play safe.

There are a lot of fantastic options available so it's just a question of having some fun exploring new ingredients and recipes. You might surprise yourself and enjoy the replacements more than what you replaced!

Know that gluten issues are a moving target, not only due to continuous new scientific findings but due to political and economical factors, and our chemically evolving food supply.

It's a controversial topic all around from what contains gluten to what are legal and "medically" safe amounts.

Unfortunately, the people declaring what are safe amounts are funded by the government... the governments are funded by large food manufacturers... *I'll let you do the math.* Legal disclaimer: that is my PERSONAL opinion. But I'll share what I have found...

I am not going to sub-phrase or re-word, I am going to print sources of studies, with their conclusions, so that you get it directly "from the horses' mouths." I am quoting directly with no expansion of my own:

Mehr S, Kakakios A, et al. **Food Protein Induced *Enterocolitis Syndrome**: 16 year experience. Pediatrics 2009; 123(3):e459-3464.

*(*enterocolitis syndrome means inflammation of the colon)*

Mehr S, Kakakios A, et al. **Rice: a common and severe cause of food protein induced *enterocolitis syndrome.** Arch Dis Child 2009;94(3):220-3.

"Maize prolamines had low but definite activity even though maize is reported to be harmless" Gut, 1983,24,825-830 *(maize is the protein in corn)*

"The allergens in rice, corn, millet, and buckwheat should be better studied before they can be recommended as alternatives for cereal allergic children." Clin Exp Allergy 1995 Nov;25(11):1100-7.

"High titres were also found...tested against wheat glutenins, albumins, and globulins, as well as against barley, oats, and maize prolamines" J Pediatr Gastroenterol Nutr. 1987 May Jun;6(3):346-50.

I could go on with scientific studies that have been published since the 80's, there are close to 20,000 studies on gluten and Celiac Disease (who knew?!) and I can tell you that there are no conclusions that are unanimous.

Please allow me to go back to my humble personal opinion, tap into your common sense, and come up with a personal conclusion of your own:

When we inject our body with "stuff" (I can't call it food) that has been genetically modified, hybridized 18 ways and back, sprayed with a chemical cocktail that targets the central nervous system of bugs and rodents *(just because humans can eat small doses of arsenic without immediately dying it doesn't make it a good idea),* and this "stuff" has no expiry date – do you think your body knows how to break that "stuff" down?

The Greeks have a word for this: "xenos" meaning "alien". The Latin "xenoliths" means strange. Alien strange food imposters, xenoestrogens affect every cell in your body and wreak havoc. *By definition they do.*

Now depending on your particular DNA, you might get cancer, your neighbor might get Alzheimer's, and I got Celiac Disease. It's as simple as that. The poisons are the same, our unique genetic codes determine our different reactions to the poisons.

When you force your body to process things it was never designed to process, expect a reaction. Expect many reactions.

And we're just talking documented and diagnosed illnesses, how about the undocumented?

Does it seem normal to you that hundreds of millions of people in developed countries are silently living with severe depression? Chronic fatigue? Chemically and biologically altered foods undoubtedly play a role, and that goes beyond gluten; now we're also talking artificial sweeteners, fillers, pesticides, fungicides; I would need to write a dozen books to list the 50,000+ chemicals in our current food supply.

That is something for you to consider. 50,000+ chemicals in our food supply!

Buy organic, support your organic farmer – they need us to create high demand so that they can make a living and maintain supply.

A quick footnote about corn and rice - and these are strictly my personal opinions, I am not telling you to eat or not eat them, I am telling you what I personally do:

CORN: I avoid it like the plague because 90%+ of corn is genetically modified (same for soy)

RICE: I occasionally eat rice, only when it is organic. Asians have lived on rice staples for centuries without creating autoimmune pandemics, so I am guessing it is our toxic bleached modified hybridized rice that we are reacting to. And I am betting it is that same standard toxic rice that they are using when they do their studies showing reactions. *...back to the evils of gluten...*

GLUTEN AND YOUR BODY

KNOWN DISORDERS LINKED TO GLUTEN

Abdominal pain

Abnormal blurred vision

ADD/ADHD

Addison's Disease

Adenocarcinoma of the intestine

Alopecia (hair loss)

Anemia

Angina Pectoris (chest pain)

Anorexia

Antiphospholipid syndrome

Anxiety

Aortic Vasculitis

Apathy

Apthous ulcers

Arthritis

Asthma

Ataxia

Atherosclerosis

Autism

Autoimmune hepatitis

Biliary cirrhosis

Bitot's spots

Blepharitis

Bone fractures

Bone pain

Bronchicctasis

Bronchoalveolitis

Cachexia

Canker Sores

Cardiomegaly

Cardiomyopathy

Cataracts

Celiac disease

Cerebral perfusion abnormalities

CFS

Cheilosis

Cholangitis

Chorea

Coagulation abnormalities

Constipation

Coronary artery disease

Crohn’s Disease

Cutaneous vasculitis

Cystic fibrosis

Decreased bone density

Delayed puberty

Dementia

Depression

Dermatitis

Dermatitis Herpetiformis

Dermatomyositis

Diabetes Mellitus type I

Diarrhea

Distention

Down's syndrome

Duodenal crosions

Dysgeusia

Dysmenorrhea

Dysphagia

Early menopause

Edema Eczema

Epilepsy

Erythema nodosum

Glossitis

Grave's Disease

H. pylori infection

Hypoglycemia

Hypospenism

IBS

Immunogglobulinopathies

Impotence

Increased risks to developing other food allergies

Infertility

Keratomalacia

Lactose intolerance

Liver and biliary tract disorders

Loss of smell

Lymphoma

Malnutrition (which leads to deficiencies, causing a myriad of other issues)

Melanoma

Mental Retardation

Migraines

Multiple sclerosis

Muscle wasting

Myopathy

Non Hodgkin lymphoma

Obesity

Osteomalacia

Osteopenia

Osteoporosis

Pancreatic insufficiency

Parathyroid carcinoma

Parkinson's

PCOS

PMS

Polyglandular syndrome

Polymyositis

Psoriasis

Seleroderma

Sjogren's syndrome

Small cell esophageal cancer

Spina bifida

Spontaneous abortion

Spontaneous nose bleeds

Steatorrhea

Stunted growth in children

Thrombocytopenia

Thyroiditis (hypothyroidism)

Transaminitis

Ulcerative colitis

UTI

Vaginitis

There are still many more "spin off" disorders, literally too many to list here, due to vitamin and mineral deficiencies caused by the malabsorption gluten reaction can create.

I would need to write volumes and volumes of books to go through each one, but any deficiency for a continuous period of time is potentially a hazard.

The body needs all essential nutrients to thrive. Take away your body's ability to absorb nutrients and you are leaving yourself vulnerable to every disease known and unknown to man. And for that reason alone the list of disease linked to gluten will only keep growing.

HOW ARE SO MANY DISORDERS POSSIBLE FROM JUST GLUTEN

When I start to talk about all the possible effects of gluten, I usually get a very confused look that says "how is that possible?"

It's a valid question. How is it possible for ONE thing to cause so many different issues and opposite issues like both weight gain AND weight loss?

Quite simply: gluten disrupts. We know it causes inflammation throughout the body and creates intestinal damage to those prone to it, causing malabsorption, thus causing weight loss. The next person might be weaker in their glands and have thyroid malfunctions, causing weight gain. Same culprit, different result.

Gluten + your specific body/DNA = unique results.

(that formula is not limited to gluten, it is all disruptors like aspartame and high fructose corn syrup)

Gluten targets cardiac, cognitive, dermatological, hepatic, musculoskeletal, and neurological systems. Once we understand that, it becomes easy to see why it can trigger hundreds of disorders. 300+ disorders according to the University of Chicago.

COMMON SYMPTOMS

Abdominal bloating and/or pain

Abnormal stools

Acidosis

Anxiety

Back pain

Bleeding gums

Blood in stool

Brain Fog

Constipation

Deficiencies (leading to many disorders, even fatality)

Dehydration (even when drinking plenty of water)

Depression

Diarrhea (often causing IBS mis-diagnosis)

Difficulty concentrating

Dry or excessively dry skin and scalp

Fatigue

Flatulence (gas)

Foul-smelling stool

Gastric bloating

Hair Loss

Headaches

Heartburn

Hives

Irritability

Joint pain

Loss of dental enamel

Migraines

Miscarriages

Mood swings

Muscle cramping

Nausea

Pale sores in the mouth

Peripheral neuropathy

Skin disorders and rashes

Tingling and numbness (check B_{12} levels)

Tooth enamel deterioration

Tremors

Vomiting

Weight gain (may trigger thyroid malfunction)

Weight loss (malnutrition)

The fact is ANY symptom could be coming from a gluten reaction; not very encouraging and all the more reason you should be tested.

The misconception is that only the intestines are affected, or that gluten causes strictly digestive disorders. The reality is that your entire body becomes collateral damage.

When you have inflammation or antibodies floating throughout your system, there is no way that the "problem area" is going to be contained to one thing.

YOU DON'T HAVE TO HAVE CELIAC DISEASE FOR GLUTEN TO MAKE YOU SICK

Here are the MOST important things you need to know about Gluten Sensitivity vs. Celiac Disease:

1) Gluten Sensitivity and Celiac are not one and the same. Celiac is just 1 of 300 disorders caused by gluten

2) They BOTH cause inflammation which leads to serious physical and neurological issues

3) The mortality rate on both is high! As a matter of fact, an important study[1] published by The Journal of the American Medical Association found that mortality rates were highest in patients with inflammation (gluten sensitivity, NOT diagnosed with Celiac) than those who were diagnosed with Celiac Disease.

The rates from that study[1] for increased mortality:
39% for those with Celiac Disease
72% for non-Celiacs with inflammation from gluten

GLUTEN SENSITIVITY CAN BE MORE FATAL THAN CELIAC DISEASE!

Okay, so what are all the terms and what's the difference between them. Here we go:

CELIAC DISEASE:

1) You need to have a specific genetic predisposition: HLA-DQ2 or HLA-DQ8 genes

2) Your intestines must show "villous atrophy" which means they have flattened and not absorbing nutrition properly *(I will rant about this insane factor in the next chapter – and it is absolute need-to-know information!)*

3) Your body generates particular antibodies when you eat gluten because it sees them as a poison and tries to defend itself by creating defense mechanisms (the antibodies).

GLUTEN SENSITIVITY:

1) You do NOT have the specific genes to qualify you to be one of the chosen few in the Celiac Club, but your body has negative reactions when you consume gluten

2) You have the genes that predispose you to Celiac Disease but your intestines have not been completely destroyed yet *(more on this shortly)*

TESTING

WHY TESTING IS CRITICAL

Call me crazy, but wouldn't you want to know what you have or don't have and what you are at most risk for so that you can do everything you can to take counter-measures?

I am hearing more and more doctors suggesting that patients just do a self-test by eliminating gluten from their diet for a few weeks and see if they feel better. Then re-introduce gluten, so if symptoms appear you'll know there's an issue, just remove gluten from your diet and don't worry about anything else. ?!?!!?

Why is that thinking wrong? Let me count the ways. First let me say, if there was a drug to prescribe, these doctors would be singing a different tune. Since the solution is strictly diet based and they can't profit from that, they are suggesting people self-diagnose and self-manage potentially fatal conditions.

An allergy is when you have an immune reaction and your body creates antibodies. **An intolerance** is a non-immune reaction but causes disruption. **Sensitivity** is a gray area in between, but causes inflammation.

Gluten intolerance causes "Gut Dysbiosis", you probably have heard the term "leaky gut". This means your body doesn't accept gluten and it can't process it, so it sits there and generates bacteria that shouldn't be in your body. That bacteria creates other elements which then cause actual tissue damage. The number of diseases you then become at high risk for are alarming.

Gluten Allergy will cause 2 types of immune reactions: "acute" (that's me, reaction 30 minutes to 3 hours) or "delayed hypersensitivity" which is really no better as far as physical damage goes. They both cause inflammation and eventual tissue damage.

So if I am at an airport and starving to death, and I am not certain if the only food I can get my hands on is gluten free or not, and no one can tell me – wouldn't it be good to know if I have a condition that leads to cancer or something that is just going to cause a skin rash for a bit?

Not to mention, if I have an acute reaction, I would rather be hungry a few hours than spend the entire flight in the tiny bathroom on the plane (including when the plane hits turbulence).

While I'm at it, I want to know if my body is generating antibodies, has t-cell reaction, could be in harm's way for 3-6 months after a 1/4 teaspoon of contamination, and on and on it goes. Don't you want to know what you are specifically dealing with?

WHERE THE MEDICAL SYSTEM FAILS, WHAT YOU NEED TO KNOW

(This chapter could easily be a 10-volume book series)
I apologize in advance if this section sounds like a rant, but really, it's hard to keep cool! I've got 3 major issues:

"VILLOUS ATROPHY" means the villi (the things inside your intestines that absorb nutrition) have sustained immense damage, flattened, you are no longer absorbing food properly and you are now at much higher risks to several diseases and fatality. Your doctor must find villous atrophy in your intestines to officially diagnose you with Celiac Disease.

Here is my problem with this: what if you have the genetic disposition, are suffering from symptoms, are physically and/or neurologically degrading, but the villi in your intestines are simply flattening at a slow speed and since the doctor doesn't see "villous atrophy" (which means total devastation), he will tell you that you don't have Celiac Disease and you are ok to eat gluten.

It's like you are driving in a tunnel, we know there's a fire at the other end, no other exits, but since your car isn't on fire itself and hasn't made contact with the fire yet you are told it is ok to keep driving in the one-way tunnel. It makes no sense to me to wait until all the damage is done before taking precautions. If you have antibodies in your system, "fire" is inevitable.

Even more maddening is that they scientifically[3] know the evolution from gluten reaction to full blown disease: mucosal inflammation, then crypt hyperplasia, and finally villous atrophy. So we watch instead of prevent.

First and foremost you want to test for the specific genes and know if you are predisposed for Celiac Disease or not. Ruling it out doesn't mean you are not sensitive to gluten but at least you will be aware one way or the other.

If you do test positive for the HLA-DQ2 or HLA-DQ8 genes, for goodness sake don't wait until you trigger Celiac Disease to eliminate gluten from your diet. It's an irreversible auto-immune disorder and it is something you do not want to live with, believe me.

It's manageable but it complicates your life. Remember my description of making a decision at the airport whether to stay hungry or not? If you wait until you trigger Celiac Disease, then you just killed your options. If you know you are predisposed but eat gluten ONLY in "emergency" kind of situations, like airports, traveling in foreign countries, the odd times when you just can't confirm gluten free or not – you are still ok. Once you awaken the dragon, those options are gone and all of the above are much harder to manage.

Ok, enough of my ranting on that. I think testing is really important, but moving on…

FALSE DIAGNOSIS

It takes an average of 11 years to diagnose Celiac Disease and anywhere from 1 to never to diagnose Gluten Sensitivity (when was the last time your doctor suggested testing for inflammation after you had a sandwich instead of prescribing an anti-depressant?)

Part of the problem has been methods of testing. For Celiac Disease the gold standard in my time was still biopsy. Unfortunately far too many doctors are today still using this method to test and declaring the person non-Celiac when they actually are a Celiac.

This happens because a biopsy is like testing for dust in a 14 room house: you take a swab from the kitchen counter and declare the house has no dust. Does that sound accurate to you? That's exactly what a biopsy does; they take swabs from an area of your intestines and determine if the villi are damaged enough to declare Celiac yet. If not, or if they "missed the spot" let's wait a few years until more damage is done to test again. It's a ludicrous negligent archaic method and I have to edit myself to not say what I really want to say!

I have met people who tested negative half a dozen times over the course of years before they finally tested positive. I met a lady who was put on anti-depressants for 21 years before realizing it was all just a gluten problem! Another on thyroid pills for 8 years. Did their health and quality of life need to suffer all that time?

RECOGNIZING SYMPTOMS

My third and final rant: I have asked several doctors and those who teach Celiac Disease in graduate school how doctors are taught to suspect gluten issues.

Are you ready for what I was told? First, do you remember the long list of symptoms listed earlier? Okay, here is what the few doctors who are even aware of gluten sensitivity are told are symptoms: bloating, diarrhea, stomach pain, vomiting, weight loss.

5 symptoms. That's f-i-v-e. *I have to edit myself again.*

Most people don't even get those 5. So what happens is that the damage is silently ongoing and the person suffers tissue damage, which leads to many other (often irreversible) diseases. It's all preventable!

Hopefully with gluten becoming a bigger and bigger problem, doctors will start to actually come up to speed on the topic on their own. Sadly, right now bloggers are better informed than the majority of doctors. And THAT is no exaggeration. A month after I was diagnosed an E.R. doctor asked me if Celiac is spelled with an "S" or a "C". *I kid you not.*

ALL this to say: if you do not feel well, demand specific testing for antibodies – do not rely on your doctor to be thorough – he or she probably has zero training on the subject of gluten.

UP TO DATE TESTING METHODS

TESTING FOR CELIAC DISEASE

First you want to do a DNA test to see if you have one or both of the genes (HLA-DQ2, HLA-DQ8) for Celiac Disease. This is done via blood test or cheek swab and completely painless.

Genetic testing can be done by your doctor and now there are even at-home kits (about $400) from a company called "Kimball Genetics and Prometheus Laboratories". You do not need to be eating gluten for genetic testing.

Having the genes doesn't mean you have Celiac Disease. It means it can be triggered at any time and you should avoid gluten to prevent that from happening. It makes complete sense to prevent an irreversible auto-immune disorder from developing if you know you are predisposed to it.

If you have the genes the next step is to test for antibodies to see if Celiac has indeed been triggered. If it has, you need to do some damage control and focus on healing and re-building your system.

WHO IS AT MOST RISK?

If someone in your immediate family (siblings, parents, or children) has Celiac Disease, your risks go up to 1 in 22. Second degree relatives like cousins and grandparents make your risk 1 in 39. So if a family member has been diagnosed, you definitely want to be screened.

FYI The latest statistics are showing that 35% of the American population has one of the genes necessary for Celiac Disease[10]. *This isn't some remote issue anymore.*

Those with European descent are at higher risk. It's interesting to note that Celiac Disease is most prevalent in "land of gluten" (Italy) per capita and they have started doing screen tests for children right in their schools.

Not at risk is one entire race: the Japanese. If you are Japanese and from a family with no mixed marriages, you cannot have the genes for Celiac Disease – but that doesn't make you immune from Gluten Sensitivity.

TESTING FOR ANTIBODIES

They are:
tTG: anti-tissue transglutaminase
EMA: anti-endomysium
DGP: anti-deamidated gliadin peptides

Usually the testing is done in reverse order: first they test for antibodies (which would show a reaction to gluten) and if there are antibodies present, the old method was to do a biopsy- which is exactly what I went through *(and what a horrendous experience).*

Testing for antibodies first is fine, but biopsy is outdated. As I mentioned earlier, it is not an accurate method, leading to a lot of "false negatives", leaving the person suffering only to come back years later to test positive.

If the antibodies are present, then you already know you are reacting to gluten; there is probably inflammation and regardless of Celiac genes (though I would want to know), you should avoid gluten as much as possible, really and truly, you should avoid gluten completely.

Since testing for anti-bodies means they are testing for a reaction to gluten, obviously that means gluten must be present.

If you suspect you are reacting to gluten, especially if you are experiencing pain and actual symptoms, I suggested you get tested immediately. That way you don't have to put yourself through the unnecessary process of clearing your system and then being forced to re-introduce gluten again so you can get tested.

Just to be totally clear: only testing for genes/DNA can be done without the presence of gluten.

All other tests will be affected, often meaning false negatives, if the person has gone gluten free even for a short period of time. So you still need to be eating gluten to do all tests outside of genetic testing.

OTHER TYPES OF TESTING

Total Serum IgA tests for IgA deficiency, which can affect accuracy of anti-body testing

EMA-IgA this is a very specific pre-screening type of test for Celiac Disease; elevated EMA means very high chances of the person having Celiac Disease. But this test is not as sensitive as the tTG-IgA; 5-10% of Celiacs test negative for EMA.

tTG-IgA this one is tricky and where many doctors fail the patient. While someone with Celiac Disease will almost always test positive for tTG, so do some people with autoimmune liver disorders, Type I Diabetes, and Hashimoto's. This can lead to a "false positive" result and leave the person dangerously open to further problems that can develop from their actual disease going untreated. **Yet another reason I urge people to get genetic testing.** ...this way if you don't have the genes for Celiac but are unwell, then you and your doctor know that something else is going on and further testing is required.

It's downright dangerous and negligent to allow people to do a little diet elimination test while there might be serious underlying issues.

BOTTOM LINE ON TESTING: insist on knowing where you stand and if your doctor disagrees, fire them, find a new one.

Imagine you have diabetes and that falsely threw off a tTG screening test, making your doctor think you have Celiac Disease – and something as serious as diabetes goes untreated…

Do not become a statistic. Testing is fast and easy nowadays. You have a right to know what's going on with your own body!

WHAT IS GLUTEN IN

HIDDEN SOURCES THAT ARE MAKING AND KEEPING YOU SICK

ARTIFICIAL FLAVOR/COLOR

Always side with caution when you see vague or general terms. Food coloring can contain many ingredients within itself. Artificial flavors and colors may or may not be safe; only the manufacturer can confirm if the product is 100% gluten free (GF). You always want specifics with food, you never want to just blindly accept vague blanket terms.

CANDY, CHOCOLATE, COUGH DROPS

Often dusted with flour to prevent sticking to the wrapping, and since the flour is not an actual ingredient IN the candy, the manufacturer usually will not list it and the loopholes in the label laws of most countries allow that to happen. Today there are so many gluten free versions of these products available; it is quite easy to substitute. Look for specific labeling indicating certified 100% gluten free, preferably from a dedicated gluten free facility if that is an option.

CHEESE

One of the most disputed topics when discussing gluten free or not... so I went in the field to do research that I know no one else did.

Most cheese is safe, but not all. Blue cheese, Chilton, Roquefort are not always safe; avoid veined cheeses or any that are coated with "mystery" products unless you have confirmed the cheese making process with that specific brand/company.

I was recently told by a U.S. "expert" that only France uses flour in veined cheese... meanwhile two summers ago I went on a wine tour through Quebec's (Canada) wine region and visited neighboring dairy farms... you guessed it, flour in their blue cheese as well as a special cranberry/port stilton. I watched them make it with my own eyes. I watched pure white flour get added to the mix along with a color preservative.

The minute there is more than just cheese, even herbs, find out what is binding those added flavors to the cheese.

Do not ever take it for granted that methods are restricted to any specific country. It's a small world and chefs move around a lot, bringing their learnt techniques with them. There is no such thing as "xyz" only happens in a certain country! Everything happens everywhere.

Also avoid pre-shredded cheeses; they can be dusted with flour to prevent sticking - too thin a coat for the naked eye to see. As with anything else you consume, check each ingredient on the label since recipes can vary and if it's a product you really love or find convenient, take the time to call the specific manufacturer and find out if their product is safe for you. It might take a few minutes to do but it will save your body from a lot of unnecessary damage.

...remember that not everyone shows symptoms, but the damage is still being done, so don't risk it.

COMMON DRINKS, COLAS, ALCOHOL

Many of them are gluten free but caution with caramel coloring, it is an ingredient made up of several others, and the recipes vary. Be on alert with root beers, and any specially flavored drinks – the honey colored drinks should raise a flag. Barley malt and wheat are common ingredients in the mix to get those brownish colors.

Distilled alcohol is generally safe, though vodka and rum manufacturers outright state their flavored products are not gluten free. Wine coolers and regular beer are definitely not gluten free, but there are gluten free versions available.

Regular wine is generally* safe (both red and white), as are champagne, port, and sherry.

**don't shoot the messenger*, I am a wine drinker too! I say "generally" only because there are some winemakers that use fining agents that contain gluten. And there are manufacturers of the oak wine barrels themselves that use flour paste when sealing the oak slabs (which I have also personally watched by a manufacturer in France). These are trace amounts, but no amount of gluten is safe for a Celiac so you may consider verifying with your favorite vintners.

CROSS-CONTAMINATION

Eating at a friend's or even hosting your own party, some simple precautions will go a long way.

Double dipping can be a catastrophe. Ask your host to put aside a little plate with a spoon or two of safe dips before any guests arrive – this will ensure that no one with regular crackers or chips will contaminate food that you might also consume.

Same rule applies to cheese; cut a few pieces of safe cheeses for yourself before substances from unsafe foods contaminate through the knives or platter or hands.

Avoid touching the bread basket when it is passed around – the flour dust can transfer easily to your hands. And please don't ever feel bad - you would happily accommodate anyone with a food intolerance and your friends will feel the same way.

Flour dust is almost invisible and if you are eating your own gluten free bread or crackers, touching the regular bread basket will cause cross contamination with your own hands. My family has gotten great with this and I even have a close friend who always jokes at dinner parties with "there goes Jaqui, doing the waltz dip at the dinner table again" (he has playfully named my backwards "duck" from the bread basket as it gets passed over me the "waltz dip"). Believe me, people will get used to little safety measures like that and it will even be something you can turn into a funny thing.

Is there something breaded going on the grill before your food? I once watched a friend tell me my eggplants were coming along wonderfully, and when I asked his wife what she uses for the burgers that the rest of the party was going to be eating she said "beef, eggs, my special family secret spices, and bread crumbs". ?!!? Bread crumbs mixed right in the burger meat, on the same grill as my eggplants... good thing the raw salad was fantastic and I actually gladly turned the eggplant into a wonderful dip for everyone else, but I didn't eat it.

DINING OUT

Good humor and asking politely will certainly go a long way, but be sure you are clear about the severity of your gluten intolerance. Your health is ultimately your responsibility.

Let's take a safe item like potatoes – if you are ordering fries, find out if other items, like breaded onion rings, are cooked in the same fryer. If so, then the oil will be contaminated. Go with baked potato and make sure it is not cooked on a grill along with other breaded items.

Asking for a bun-less burger? Great. It might not be enough though. Ask if everyone else's buns are being warmed on the same grill. Is breaded chicken being cooked on the same grill as your meat?

When you are eating out the danger zones are not just ingredients IN the food, they are cooking processes, contaminated spatulas and hands, shared cooking surfaces, marinades, sauces, spices...

Gluten awareness is thankfully rising, but don't take it for granted that people understand the topic thoroughly. Most restaurants just know that breads, pastas, and cookies/cakes are on the danger list – you would be shocked at how many have heard of gluten, confidently tell you they can accommodate, but they have never heard the term "cross-contamination".

Always ask the detailed questions you need to ask to gauge if they really have a good policy in place or if they are just trying to win the gluten customer share.

I hate to say it, but a lot of people are seeing gluten as a food fad and have no understanding of the serious medical implications. Whether they are greedy or ignorant, the damage to you will be the same.

Whether eating out or at a friend's, never be shy to ask questions about preparation, seasoning, and cooking tools. Consider things like gravy (usually thickened with flour). Take time to consider typical toppings or side dishes that may make an otherwise safe dish, unsafe.

I've seen protein mixes that gyms use in their smoothies containing barley or coloring that include malt and how do I know this? I am not shy, when in doubt I ask the bartender "can I please see that container of protein mix you are using?" and I read the label. It's MY health and due diligence is not an option.

DRIED GOODS

The risk of cross-contamination is high when it comes to certain safe foods like beans and lentils because the manufacturers that produce/package these products usually also produce flour and other foods with gluten.

Have you ever seen the inside of these processing plants? The employees are all in astronaut suits (I'm not being dramatic, they are) and it is because flour flies. Powder flies. They wouldn't be able to breathe. So if the beans are on one assembly line and wheat flour is nearby...

Now I can't talk about this without mentioning the law. As of 2012 the United States has no official policy, they have a "proposed law" that the FDA is looking at. Canada on the other hand has had laws in place for a few years and are being applauded by the Celiac communities. **I seem to be the only person who actually read the Canadian Government's official policy.** IT DOES NOT ACCOUNT FOR CROSS-CONTAMINATION. Sorry to yell in capitals but I wish I could yell it from rooftops... let me explain...

A company needs to be below 20ppm (part per million) of gluten in the product and they can legally label it gluten free. Those 20ppm's do NOT take into consideration any flour that might be flying over from the next assembly line. This means there could be a 63,546ppm's in the official "gluten free" product and it is still legally labeled gluten free. Remember the astronaut suits? Great law. Unbelievable. But that's the reality. That loophole allows for ANY amount of gluten to be in a product.

"Buyer beware", your government is not there to protect you. They are there to protect major food companies.

Ideally you want to buy your dried goods from a company that specifically says they are a Gluten-Free Dedicated Facility. That's your best option.

If that's not possible then you really want to make sure you do a great job of washing your dried goods thoroughly before using them. Put on your paranoia hat here and wash over and over to get every last trace amount that the naked eye can't see off.

GLUTEN FREE AND WHEAT FREE ARE NOT THE SAME

Gluten comes in many forms – check individual ingredients. "Wheat free" alone is not safe. There are millions of boxes with a 50 year shelf life on grocery shelves that say "wheat free" and they were manufactured before gluten became a hot topic, so be aware of this differentiation.

GRAS (GENERALLY RECOGNIZED AS SAFE)

Caution with the term "harmless level of gluten". There is no such thing as a harmless level of gluten.

GROCERY GUIDES

They can misguide you because manufacturers regularly change their ingredients. Numerous items that were safe at the time the guide was published might not be safe just months later. These guides are updated once a year at best, once every 3-4 years on average and they are usually geographically contained.

Local manufacturers are being e-mailed or called and asked about the gluten content of their product, and just like the U.S. based cheese "expert" who said only France uses flour in cheese… while a short hop north of the border I know for a fact there are Quebec cheese makers also using flour… this is a dangerous thing if U.S. companies start assuming some of their imported products are safe.

Remember that corn might be king in The United States, but wheat rules in Canada (and many other countries) and Canada ships 40% of its products to the U.S. There are 35,000+ trucks a DAY shipping everything from paper products to, yes, food… much of which contains wheat.

The cheese example is one, and the maltodextrin example is also perfect to mention here: the U.S. uses mainly corn to make maltodextrin, Canada uses mostly wheat.

By law, labels must always be changed when ingredients change, so the only truly safe route is to always check every ingredient on every label, which is why grocery guides are a hidden danger to you, as well as unverified ingredients within an ingredient.

Use the A to Z list in this book to ensure safety.

GROUND SPICE

Buy spices in their whole form and grind at home (this also tastes so much better). Inexpensive coffee or spice grinders make it so simple.

Besides the fact that pre-ground spices comprise risks of fillers and cross contamination, you might also be consuming harmful toxins.

A simple example: table salts are bleached for a brighter white color; this is done with a harmful chemical that goes unnoticed since we consume salt in small doses.

Good salt options are pure Himalayan or gray sea salt, it may cost you an extra few dollars a year – this is such a nominal amount, yet the cumulative effect of several minor changes will be significant.

INGREDIENTS WITHIN AN INGREDIENT

This is when an ingredient in food is made up of several other ingredients. So if it takes 5 different grains or seeds or starches to make up the 1 ingredient listed, we need to know what those 5 things are.

"Ingredients within an ingredient" is a concept that is important to understand because it is often a source of hidden gluten.

Our perfect example is maltodextrin; can be made with wheat, potato, or corn – there is no way to know which starch the manufacturer used unless they have specified it on the label (which is something you will not see often), so it needs to be verified and avoided until confirmed as GF.

KISSING

...talk about a source no one thinks about! Saliva. Yes, I learned this one the hard way. If you are a little sensitive or are avoiding gluten by choice and not for medical allergy or intolerance, you're fine.

If you have Celiac Disease or know you are extra sensitive and react to small amounts of gluten, make sure your loved one brushes their teeth AND rinses with a GF mouthwash before kissing you if they have eaten foods containing gluten (including drinking beer).

KITCHEN CARE

Get two cutting boards and make sure they are different materials to avoid mix-ups or residual matter; glass for gluten free and wood for standard (wood tends to trap substance even after washed).

Keep the standard food, utensils, toaster, on bottom shelves to keep crumbs from falling onto gluten free shelves. Same for refrigerator and cupboards – dedicate all the top shelves for gluten free items.

Do not wipe crumbs from counters with the same towels that you might also use to dry plates. Color coding is very helpful here: green (go) =gluten free, red (stop) =gluten.

Use different colored containers to store gluten free food. Keep two sets of colors to avoid mix-ups. If you can find them in green and red to keep it consistent, great. If not, no problem! Get green and red stickers or green and red markers.

Tape "GF" stickers onto peanut butter jars, butter, and all other foods prone to double dipping or spreading onto bread; dedicate one set to remain gluten free. If someone spread peanut butter onto regular bread, went back in the jar with that contaminated knife and scooped out a bit more – your eye might not catch those crumbs the next day. You don't want to worry about things like that. A dedicated gluten free jar with a clear sticker makes it safer for the Celiac and easier on the entire household.

A PERSONAL NOTE - I repeat this because I know how hard it is at first... *Do not be discouraged,* these are all things that need to be set up just once, soon they will be second nature for you and your family. The more care you take in setting up a full list of the safety measures listed here, the more you guarantee that you will avoid accidental contamination.

MEAT GLUE

Those two words should never be together, yet astonishingly, they are together and in your grocery store. The "glue" is "transglutaminase enzyme", which is 100% gluten and used to "glue" small pieces of meat together to be sold to you as one larger piece. Watch the video titled "meat glue" on my YouTube channel (Jaqui Karr TV) in my "gluten playlist". Be sure to subscribe to my channel to get important updates!

Buy from an organic farmer if possible, or whole pieces that are unmistakably unaltered from their original form. If you find these too expensive I strongly suggest you cut back on meat consumption and when you do buy meat, make it a quality (and safe) product.

MEDICATION

Our focus is usually on food alone, especially when newly diagnosed, but *EVERY* single thing we digest must be checked. Unfortunately, your doctor will usually not know which medication is gluten free – but pharmacists can find out for you.

Again, I don't trust outdated lists printed every few years. Your safer bet is asking your pharmacist.

MODIFIED – *ANYTHING*

The term "modified food" or "modified x product", like corn starch, is very vague and unsafe. "Modified" can mean anything. It can be maddening (hopefully maddening enough to get you to send your local politician a letter to demand for 100% transparent food labeling) but again, your health is your responsibility.

Do not assume your government has you covered. Your government has their donators covered, which are often major food manufacturers who demand for loopholes the size of the Pacific Ocean so they can keep costs low and profits high. The real cost is the consumer's health, *but I'll stop talking.*

NATURAL FLAVOR & COLOR

Do not let the word “natural” misguide you; *wheat is a natural product…*

Always be careful with vague and general terms. You want to know EXACTLY what you are eating; this is another example of possible ingredients within an ingredient. Find out exactly what substances are in every food.

NON-FOOD ITEMS

Cosmetics (particularly lipstick, lip balm) chewing gum, breath mints, toothpaste, mouthwash, envelopes and stamps (buy self-sealing, don’t lick the glue on stamps/envelopes); Play-Doh is a surprising one – and we know how often kids put their hands in their mouth (or grab a cookie), so if your child is gluten sensitive, be sure to get rid of Play-Doh.

Remember that your skin is your largest organ and its pores absorb easily. If you do not want something IN your body, do not put it ON your body.

Look at everything you will digest or your skin will absorb with a sharper eye, and when in doubt – avoid or replace it.

RAW or HOME MADE VERSIONS

Of course going raw will ensure absolute safety, but it is not easy or convenient for most people. Even if not a completely raw diet, try to go to raw forms with as much as possible: i.e. homemade pesto instead of from a jar. You can't imagine how much better homemade salad dressings taste, and most will keep for over a week. Ketchup, SO easy to make and completely incomparable to the store bought stuff.

Scan your pantry and refrigerator and make a list of things that can be made naturally at home with just a few extra minutes. "Like" my facebook page called "NakedFood" for fantastic ideas and recipes.

ROASTED NUTS

I have visited nut distributors who roast on site and discovered that many of them put a half teaspoon of wheat flour into the machine before they start to "dry roast" and this prevents the nuts from sticking to each other when packaged. They put slightly more with specially flavored ones.

It's not an absolute, there are roasters who do not do this, but many do – so again it is a question of being aware of the process and asking questions before you buy. If you see sesame seeds and caramel flavor on almonds ask what is “binding” the sesame seeds to the almonds. *They don’t stick on their own.*

Keep in mind the retailer will not always know. If you see a puzzled or blank look even for a second, be sure to take it one level up. Get to the wholesaler or manufacturer... someone who actually knows the manufacturing process for a fact and is familiar with the facility that the specific food in question is coming from, and confirm with them whether this product is completely gluten free or not.

Processing methods are important to understand. Not fun, but necessary. And remember, do not trust a blanket method. Chef techniques vary and so do manufacturing processes.

Some companies have machines that are decades old and it would cost millions to replace them. So while one manufacturer with a brand new facility might make cookies one way, another manufacturer with 55 year old machines might be making it a whole other way. You want specifics by brand and facility/company.

Long before the word “gluten” was in the dictionary, wheat was considered “the staff of life” and a lot of food processes have centered around wheat for the past century (which might be a clue as to why Celiac Disease exploded 400% in less than two generations).

"SAFE" FOODS

Be aware of seasoning, coloring, flavoring, marinades. The obvious may be simple: "avoid bread and pizza". Watch for the not-so-obvious like wheat in ice cream, barley in sauces and dressings, malt in chocolate, wheat in soy sauce....

I once has a client who didn't seem to be getting well and swore she was 100% gluten free; I raided her kitchen to find a half dozen products containing gluten, like barley in the Worcestershire sauce she was marinating her meat in, malt in her chocolate cocoa mix, barley in one of her teas, and her shampoo had "wheat germ oil" in huge print right on the bottle... which she was massaging into her scalp daily as well as absorbing it via skin as she washed it off her hair.

Clearly she hadn't quite grasped the concept of "check every ingredient on every label of everything you come into contact with".

People know gluten is a protein in certain grains, but our highly industrialized food supply is a mystery to most of us. We have no idea what is going into processed foods. Recently more information has been coming to the surface, such as the hundreds of variations used with corn and sugar, keep in mind there are thousands of variations with gluten – it won't always be as obvious as bread and pasta.

SUSHI

Very high risk of cross contamination with breaded, fried, tempura foods. Have you EVER seen a sushi chef soap his hands between rolls? Never. The restaurant would come to a dead halt and go out of business.

He might wipe his hands (on the same towel over and over), but he's not removing gluten from them and he's certainly not removing gluten from the mat he's using to roll.

My second concern, after cross-contamination, is the nori sheets themselves. They SHOULD be 100% seaweed, but the cheaper quality are not and many countries, especially in Asia, that make them often use barley and wheat as fillers and binders.

There is also a major health concern outside of gluten (if you are eating sushi with fish and not just vegetables); it is best explained in the extraordinary documentary "The Cove". "Mercury Rising" in the special features section discusses concerns with the toxic mercury levels in fish; *highly recommended* to watch this movie for both human and cetacean health.

...all this said, I often find myself gravitating to sushi bars when stuck in an airport a long time. I explain my severe intolerance to the chef and simply get them to give me plain rice from the cooker (not the outside batch he keeps using his hands to grab from), and a bunch of the ingredients (carefully chopped on a clean surface) that they use inside their rolls. Tedious? Maybe. *But I like traveling without cramps.*

The better option is to prepare ahead and pack food, but you can't always foresee a 12 hour unexpected layover.

TEA

Many contain unsafe flavoring products, check labels carefully. There is a risk of cross contamination during the packaging process since most tea producers offer varieties of flavors.

Tea is also an item where vague terms such as "natural flavors" are found often. Whenever possible, buy whole leaf teas, otherwise verify with the manufacturer if there are vague terms in the ingredients.

A special note regarding Genmaicha tea (Japanese green tea with toasted brown rice): there are some manufacturers making this with roasted barley instead of rice. The roasting/toasting process might not make it so easy to differentiate whether you are seeing barley or rice, so be sure to verify.

VINEGAR

Apple cider, distilled, wine, balsamic are usually safe (unless extra flavoring or coloring has been added, then it needs to be verified).

White vinegar might not be; the manufacturer can use wheat, rye or barley in their process and non-distilled probably contains gluten.

If you do not have clear information, avoid it. Very inexpensive white vinegar should raise an alert flag and should be verified. So in the case of food containing vinegar as an ingredient, using common sense: if an entire box of that food retails at $1.99, do you suppose they are springing for the expensive distilled vinegar or the non-distilled cheaper kind?

Please do not listen to the "experts" (I have even seen an M.D. claim all vinegar is safe)... they clearly haven't put on the lab coat and visited a food manufacturer and asked detailed questions.

+++++

This can all be overwhelming,

I'm really very aware because I have Celiac Disease myself and when I first got sick, my reaction was much worse and much more extreme than 99% of the average cases. Believe me when I say *"I know what you are going through".*

However, BECAUSE I had such a hard time with it, it forced me to look at things a lot more carefully and closely than everyone else – including the outright reckless M.D.'s who know nothing about food processing and who have never felt that distinct intestinal cramp themselves.

A lot of this is mindset - no different from everything else in life. Your attitude towards this whole adventure will make all the difference in the world. Notice the reference to it as an adventure and not anything restrictive. If you moved to a foreign country and did not have access to the foods you are used to, you would undoubtedly adjust and enjoy new tastes. This is an opportunity for you to discover new foods and great new recipes.

There are wonderful ways to make your favorites with completely natural gluten free ingredients from pizza crusts to olive bread! A lot of great gluten free food has been hitting the grocery shelves lately so enjoy the exploration of a whole new world of food!

Just be mindful that gluten free doesn't mean healthy, there are a lot of safe foods that are still toxic from an overall health perspective – you don't want extreme high levels of sugar or synthetic sweeteners that your body doesn't know how to process.

Stay Safe!

THE A TO Z SHOPPING LIST

Always check every ingredient on every label; it is the ONLY way to ensure safety

---

IMPORTANT TO READ: "all grains" discussion at the beginning of this book in the "what is gluten" section

S=Safe

N=Not safe

?=investigate/caution

N-Abyssinian Hard (wheat triticum durum)
S-Acacia Gum
S-Acesulfame K
S-Acesulfame Potassium
S-Acetanisole
S-Acetic Acid
S-Acetic Anhydride
S-Acetolactate Decarboxylase
S-Acetone
S-Acetone Peroxide
S-Acetophenone
N-Acidophilus Milk
S-Acorn Quercus

S-Active Bacterial Cultures
S-Adipic Acid
S-Adzuki Bean
S-Agar
S-Agave
S-Alant Starch
S-Albumen
?-Alcohol:

SAFE: Distilled alcohol [unflavored gin, rum, vodka, whiskey], champagne, port, sherry, wine*. (*note: some winemakers use fining agents that contain gluten, plus there are manufacturers of the oak wine barrels themselves that use flour paste when sealing the oak slabs-which I have personally watched by a manufacturer in France. You may consider verifying with your favorite vintners).

NOT SAFE: Specially flavored rum, vodka, premixes, beer, wine coolers. Sake contains Koji, which may contain barley. Cider may contain barley enzymes. As with food, if all the ingredients haven't been verified or are unavailable, refrain until you can verify with manufacturer or find a gluten free substitute

N-Ale
S-Alfalfa
S-Algae
S-Algin
S-Alginate
S-Alginic Acid
S-Alkalized Cocoa

S-Alkanet
S-Allicin
S-Allura Red
S-Almond
S-Alpha-amylase
S-Alpha-lactalbumin
S-Alpha-tocopherol Acetate
S-Aluminum (gluten free but toxic in other ways)
S-Amaranth (caution with cross contamination)
S-Ambergris
S-Ammonium Alginate
S-Ammonium Bicarbonate or Carbonate
S-Ammonium Carrageenan
S-Ammonium Chloride
S-Ammonium Citrate
S-Ammonium Furcelleran
S-Ammonium Hydroxide
S-Ammonium Persulphate
S-Ammonium Phosphate
S-Ammonium Sulphate
N-Amp-Isostearoyl Hydrolyzed Wheat Protein
S-Amylase
S-Amylopectin
S-Amylose
S-Anise
S-Annatto
?-Annatto Color (multiple processing methods)

S-Anthocyanins
S-Apple Cider Vinegar
S-Arabic Gum
S-Arabinogalactan
?-Arborio Rice (see “all grains”)
S-Arrowroot (pure arrowroot is safe; commercially prepared arrow biscuits usually contain gluten)
?-Artificial Butter Flavor (recipes/ingredients vary)
?-Artificial Color (vague)
?-Artificial Flavor (vague)
N-Asafoetida (spice, often contains flour)
S-Ascorbic Acid
S-Aspartame (gluten free, but highly toxic)
S-Aspartic Acid
S-Aspic
S-Astragalus Gummifer
N-Atta Flour
S-Autolyzed Yeast Extract
?-Avena Sativa (oats - see “all grains”)
?-Avenin (see “all grains”)
S-Avidin
S-Azodicarbonamide (gluten free, but toxic)
S-Bacon (caution flavoring/spices)
S-Bacterial Cultures
?-Baking Powder (verify which starch is used)
?-Baking Soda (verify all ingredients, not all are safe)
S-Balsamic Vinegar
N-Barley
N-Barley Grass

N-Barley Hordeum Vulgare
N-Barley Malt
?-Basmati Rice (see "all grains")
S-Beans (rinse well before using, many companies packaging beans also package wheat/barley/etc and there could be a risk of cross contamination)
N-Beer
S-Beeswax
S-Bengal Gram
S-Benzoic Acid
S-Benzoyl Peroxide
S-Benzyl Alcohol
S-Besan bean (chickpea)
S-Beta Carotene
?-Beta Glucan (oats - see "all grains")
S-Betaine
S-BHA
S-BHT
S-Bicarbonate of Soda
S-Biotin
?-Black Rice (see "all grains")
N-Bleached Flour
?-Blue Cheese (may contain flour in the mold)
N-Bouillon
S-Bovine Rennet
N-Bran
N-Bread Flour
?-Brewer's Rice (see "all grains")
N-Brewer's Yeast

?-Brie Cheese (caution with coating)
S-Bromelain
S-Brominated Vegetable Oil (gluten free, often in colas, toxic in high amounts and banned in many countries)
N-Broth (many GF versions available)
N-Brown Flour
S-Brown Rice Syrup (see "all grains")
S-Brown Sugar
S-Buckwheat (risk of cross contamination, try to buy from a GF dedicated facility)
N-Bulgur
S-Butter (unflavored, check ingredients)
?-Buttermilk (most contain modified food starch)
N-Butterscotch
S-Butylated Hydroxyanisole
S-Butylated Hydroxytoluene
S-Butyl Compounds
S-Caffeine
S-Calcium Acetate
S-Calcium Alginate
S-Calcium Aluminum Silicate
S-Calcium Ascorbate
S-Calcium Carbonate
S-Calcium Carrageenan
?-Calcium Caseinate (contains MSG)
S-Calcium Chloride
S-Calcium Citrate
S-Calcium Disodium
S-Calcium Fumarate

S-Calcium Furcelleran
S-Calcium Gluconate
S-Calcium Glycerophosphate
S-Calcium Hydroxide
S-Calcium Hypophosphite
S-Calcium Iodate
S-Calcium Lactate
S-Calcium Pantothenate
S-Calcium Peroxide
S-Calcium Phosphate
S-Calcium Propionate
S-Calcium Silicate
S-Calcium Sorbate
S-Calcium Stearate
S-Calcium Stearoyl Lactylate
S-Calcium Sulfate
S-Calcium Tartrate
?-Calrose Rice (see "all grains")
?-Camembert Cheese (caution with coating)
S-Camphor (gluten free, poisonous in large amounts)
?-Candy (often dusted with flour to prevent sticking)
S-Cane Sugar
S-Cane Vinegar
S-Canola Oil (also called rapeseed oil. made from the seed of rape - which is in the grass family. tested as safe but many Celiacs have adverse reactions. Canola is often a genetically modified product that your body doesn't process well and has toxic properties. I highly recommend completely avoiding canola. Use olive oil)

S-Canthaxanthin
S-Caprylic Acid
?-Caramel Color (often made with barley malt, manufacturer must confirm ingredients used)
S-Caraway Seeds
S-Carbonated Water
S-Carbon Dioxide
S-Carboxymethyl Cellulose
S-Carmine
S-Carnauba Wax
S-Carob Bean
S-Carob Bean Gum
S-Carob Flour
S-Carrageenan
S-Carrageenan Chondrus Crispus
S-Casein
S-Cassava Manihot Esculenta
S-Castor Oil
S-Catalase
S-Cellulase
S-Cellulose
S-Cellulose Ether
S-Cellulose Gum
N-Cereal Binding
S-Cetyl Alcohol
S-Cetyl Stearyl Alcohol
S-Champagne Vinegar
S-Channa (chickpea)

S-Charcoal
?-Cheese (not all are safe, check the labels carefully; blue and veined cheese may contain trace amounts of flour, also avoid pre-shredded cheeses as they are usually coated with flour to avoid sticking or clumping)
S-Chestnuts
S-Chia
S-Chicken (fresh is safe; caution with pre-seasoned)
S-Chickpea
S-Chicory (caution if it's a coffee replacement, they often have barley and other unsafe additives)
S-Chlorella
S-Chlorine
S-Chloropentafluoroethane
S-Chlorophyll
?-Chocolate (usually unsafe, also many bars are dusted with flour to avoid sticking to wrapping)
?-Chocolate Liquor (look for added ingredients)
S-Cholecalciferol
S-Choline Chloride
N-Chorizo (usually contain cereal fillers, avoid if you don't have detailed label or verify with manufacturer)
N-Chow Mein Noodles
S-Chromium Citrate
S-Chymosin
?-Citric Acid (verify source used)
?-Clarifying Agents (may be hydrolyzed wheat)
N-Club Wheat (triticum aestivum subspecies compactum)

S-Cochineal
S-Cocoa (verify it is pure cocoa)
S-Cocoa Butter
S-Coconut
S-Coconut Flour
S-Coconut Oil
S-Coconut Vinegar
S-Coffee (thought to be safe, though many Celiacs are sensitive – possibly to a specific protein in coffee. Careful with flavors added when buying lattes or flavored milk; also be careful when buying "mocha" which is never just chocolate, there are barley additives or some other gluten to "hold" the flavor)
S-Collagen
S-Colloidal Silicon Dioxide
N-Common Wheat (Triticum aestivum)
S-Confectioner's Glaze or Sugar
?-Converted® Rice (see "all grains")
?-Cooking Spray (many contain grain or flour alcohol)
S-Copernicia Cerifera
S-Copper Sulphate
?-Corn and all by-products (see "all grains")
S-Cortisone
S-Cotton Seed
S-Cotton Seed Oil
N-Couscous
S-Cowitch
S-Cowpea
N-Cracker Meal

N-Criped Rice
S-Crospovidone
N-Croutons
S-Curcumin
S-Curds
S-Curry (pure curry safe; paste may contain gluten)
N-Custard
S-Cyanocobalamin
S-Cyclamate
S-Cysteine, L
S-Dal or Dahl (lentils)
S-D-Alpha-tocopherol
S-Dasheen Flour (taro)
S-Dates (may be coated to prevent sticking)
S-D-Calcium Pantothenate
S-Delactosed Whey (pure whey safe; altered versions may contain gluten)
?-Della Rice (see "all grains")
S-Demineralized Whey (pure whey safe; altered versions may contain gluten)
S-Desamidocollagen
S-Dextran
?-Dextrate (may be from any starch)
?-Dextri-maltose (wheat barley may be used)
?-Dextrin (can be made from wheat, corn, or several other grains)
S-Dextrose
S-Dhal
S-Dhalin

S-Dichloromethane
S-Diglyceride (unmodified)
S-Dimethylpolysiloxane Formulations
N-Dinkle (Spelt)
S-Dioctyl Sodium
S-Dioctyl Sodium Solfosuccinate
S-Dipotassium Phosphate
S-Disodium EDTA
S-Disodium Guanylate
S-Disodium Inosinate
S-Disodium Phosphate
N-Disodium Wheatgermamido Peg-2 Sulfosuccinate
S-Distilled Alcohol (distillation process makes it safe; caution with added flavors, additives, color)
S-Distilled Vinegar (see "vinegar")
S-Dry Roasted Nuts (risk of cross contamination, flour may be added to avoid clumping)
N-Durum Wheat (Triticum durum)
S-Dutch Processed Cocoa
?-Edible Coatings/Films (may be corn or wheat)
N-Edible Starch
S-EDTA (ethylenediaminetetraacetic acid)
S-Eggs
N-Einkorn (Triticum monococcum)
S-Elastin
N-Emmer (Triticum dicoccon)
N-Emulsifiers (most contain gluten)
N-Enriched Flour

N-Enzymes (may contain binders)
S-Epichlorohydrin
S-Ergocalciferol
S-Erthorbic Acid
S-Erythritol
S-Erythrosine
S-Ester Gum
S-Ethanol
S-Ethoxyquin
S-Ethyl Alcohol
S-Ethylenediaminetetraacetic Acid
S-Ethyl Maltol
S-Ethyl Vanillin
S-Expeller Pressed Canola Oil (see Canola)
N-Farina
N-Farina Graham
N-Farro
S-Fava Bean
S-Fennel
S-Ferric Orthophosphate
S-Ferrous Fumerate
S-Ferrous Gluconate
S-Ferrous Lactate
S-Ferrous Sulfate
S-Feta Cheese
N-Filler (too vague, often wheat)
S-Fish (caution with breaded, pre-seasoned, fried)
?-Flaked Rice (see "all grains")

?-Flavoring (vague term)
S-Flax
N-Flour (standard type is wheat)
S-Flour Salt
S-Folacin
S-Folate
S-Folic Acid
?-Food Coloring (vague)
?-Food Starch (can be wheat or mixture)
S-Formaldehyde (gluten free, but toxic)
S-Fructose
S-Fructose Syrup (unflavored, for corn/corn fructose see "all grains")
S-Fruit (if dried, verify for additives)
S-Fruit Juice Concentrate
S-Fruit Vinegar
N-Fu (dried wheat gluten)
S-Fumaric Acid
S-Furcelleran
S-Galactose
?-Gamma Oryzanol (verify starch used)
S-Garbanzo Beans
S-Garlic
S-Gelatin
?-Gelatinized Starch (verify type of starch)
S-Gellan Gum
?- Genmaicha Tea (sometimes made with barley instead of rice)
N-Germ

N-German Wheat
N-Gliadin
S-Glucanase
S-Glucoamylase
S-Gluconic Acid
S-Glucono Lactone (Glucono-Delta)
S-Glucose
S-Glucose Isomerase
S-Glucose Oxidase
?-Glucose Syrup (can be corn or wheat; usually listed as safe because the wheat forms are trace amounts. regardless of PPM level, *any* amount of gluten is not safe for a Celiac)
S-Glutamate
?-Glutamic Acid (MSG, can be from several grains)
?-Glutamine - glutamine & L-glutamine are the same: SAFE if the source is from animal protein or vegetable; UNSAFE when derived from wheat, peptide or bonded
N-Glutamine Peptide (usually derived from wheat)
N-Gluten
N-Glutenin
N-Gluten Peptides
?-Glutinous Rice (see "all grains", but "glutinous" with rice does not mean "gluten")
?-Glycerides (modified versions may contain wheat, unmodified are just fats and are safe)
S-Glycerin
S-Glycerol Diacetate
S-Glycerol Monoacetate

S-Glycerol Monooleate
S-Glyceryl Triacetate
S-Glyceryl Tributyrate
S-Glycine
S-Glycol
S-Glycolic Acid
S-Glycol Monosterate
N-Gorgonzola Cheese
N-Graham Flour
S-Gram flour (chick peas)
N-Granary Flour (may be combination of grains)
S-Grape Skin Extract
N-Gravy (usually thickened with wheat flour or corn starch)
?-Grits (corn – see "all grains")
N-Groats (barley, wheat)
?-Ground Spices (cross contamination/filler risk)
S-Guaiaca Gum
S-Guar Gum (guaran, can have IBS effect)
S-Gum Acacia
S-Gum Arabic
?-Gum Base (manufacturer must confirm source)
S-Gum Benzoin
S-Gum Guaiacum
S-Gum Tragacanth
N-Hard Wheat
N-Heeng
S-Hemicellulase
S-Hemp (caution with cross contamination)

S-Herbs (look for pure, many have fillers)
S-Herb Vinegar
S-Hexane (gluten free, but toxic)
S-Hexanedioic Acid
?-High Fructose Corn Syrup (see “all grains”)
N-Hing
S-Hominy
S-Honey
S-Hops
N-Hordein
N-Hordeum Vulgare Extract
S-Horseradish (safe if pure)
N-HPP
?-Hulls (outer layer of any grain, vague)
N-HVP
S-Hyacinth Bean
S-Hydrochloric Acid
N-Hydrogenated Corn Starch
N-Hydrogenated Starch Hydrolysate
S-Hydrogenated Vegetable Oil
S-Hydrogen Peroxide
S-Hydrolyzed Caseinate
S-Hydrolyzed Meat Protein
?-Hydrolyzed Oat Protein (may contain wheat)
?-Hydrolyzed Plant Protein (may contain wheat)
S-Hydrolyzed Soy Protein
?-Hydrolyzed Vegetable Protein (may contain wheat)
N-Hydrolyzed Wheat Gluten

N-Hydrolyzed Wheat Protein Pg-Propyl Silanetriol
N-Hydrolyzed Wheat Starch
S-Hydroxylated Lecithin
S-Hydroxypropyl Cellulose
S-Hydroxypropyl Methylcellulose
N-Hydroxypropyltrimonium Hydrolyzed Wheat Protein
S-Hypromellose
?-Ice Cream (check ingredients, most have gluten)
S-Illepe
S-Indian Ricegrass seed (Montina)
S-Indigotine
S-Inulin
S-Inulinase
S-Invertase
S-Invert Sugar
S-Iodine
S-Irish Moss Gelose
S-Iron Ammonium Citrate
S-Iron Oxide
S-Isinglass
S-Iso-Ascorbic Acid
S-Isobutane
S-Isolated Soy Protein
S-Isomalt
S-Isopropanol
S-Isopropyl Alcohol
?-Japonica Rice (see “all grains”)
S-Job's Tears (Hato Mugi, Juno's Tears, River Grain)
?-Jowar (Sorghum, see “all grains”)

N-Kafirin
N-Kamut (pasta wheat)
S-Karaya Gum
S-Kasha (Russian Kasha may contain millet and oats)
S-K-Carmine Color
N-Kecap Manis (soy sauce)
S-Kelp
S-Keratin
S-Ketchup (check ingredients, many unsafe)
N-Ketjap Manis (soy sauce)
S-K-Gelatin
N-Kluski Pasta
?-Koji (verify starch used)
S-Konjac
?-Koshihikari (rice – see "all grains")
S-Kudzu
S-Kudzu Root Starch
S-Lactalbumin Phosphate
S-Lactase
S-Lactic Acid
S-Lactitol
S-Lactobacillus Acidophilus
S-Lactobacillus Bifidus
N-Lacto globulin
S-Lactose (many Celiacs are lactose intolerant; reaction generally improves after adhering to GF diet for some time. I recommend coconut or a nut milk like almond milk whether the person has lactose intolerance or not)

S-Lactulose
S-Lactylic Esters of fatty acids
S-Lanolin
S-Lard
S-L-Cysteine
S-Lecithin (soy sensitive for some Celiacs)
S-Lecithin Citrate
S-Legumes
S-Lemon Grass
S-Lentils
?-L-Glutamine (see glutamine)
S-Licorice Candy or Extract (check with manufacturer)
S-Lipase
S-Lipoxidase
?-Liquor (see alcohol)
S-L-Leucine
S-L-Lysine
S-L-Methionine
S-Locust Bean Gum
S-L-Tryptophan
S-Lysozyme
N-Macha Wheat (triticum aestivum)
S-Magnesium Aluminum Silicate
S-Magnesium Carbonate
S-Magnesium Chloride
S-Magnesium Citrate
S-Magnesium Fumerate
S-Magnesium Hydroxide
S-Magnesium Oxide

S-Magnesium Phosphate
S-Magnesium Silicate
S-Magnesium Stearate
S-Magnesium Sulphate
N-Maida (Indian wheat flour)
?-Maize (corn – see "all grains")
S-Malic Acid
N-Malt
N-Malt Chocolate
N-Malted Barley Flour
N-Malted Milk
N-Malt Extract
N-Malt Flavoring
N-Maltitol (usually listed as safe because process is supposed to remove gluten from the wheat starch – trace amounts will always be left)
?-Maltodextrin (can be made from wheat, potato, rice or corn. listed as safe on most GF lists because it is a highly processed product, so assumption is gluten is removed even with wheat versions, but trace amounts may be left on product; not safe unless potato)
S-Maltol
N-Maltose (listed as safe on most lists because the manufacturing process is said to remove the gluten from end product; trace amounts or more may be left)
N-Malt Syrup
N-Malt Vinegar
S-Manganese Sulfate
S-Manioc

S-Mannitol
S-Maple Syrup (pure, unflavored)
S-Margarine (check all ingredients)
?-Masa Farina (cornstarch, see “all grains”; be cautious of “Masa de trigo”, it is wheat, not corn)
?-Masa Flour
?-Masa Harina
N-Matza
N-Matzah
N-Matzo
N-Matzo Semolina
S-Meat (watch for fillers, flavoring; try to buy full pieces and spice/marinade yourself)
S-Medium Chain Triglycerides
S-Menhaden Oil
N-Meringue
N-Meripro 711
S-Methanol
S-Methyl Alcohol
S-Methyl Cellulose
S-Methyl Paraben
S-Microcrystalline Cellulose
S-Micro-Particulated Egg White Protein
S-Milk (technically safe, but many Celiacs sensitive – see “lactose”. Caution if flavored; malted milk not safe)
S-Milk Protein Isolate (see milk or lactose)
?-Millet (see “all grains”)
N-Milo (Sorghum)

S-Mineral Oil
S-Mineral Salts
N-Mir
N-Mirin (many brands contain wheat)
N-Miso (contains barley)
N-Modified Corn Starch (see "all grains" & vague)
?-Modified Food Starch (caution, vague term)
S-Molasses (unflavored)
S-Molybdenum Amino Acid Chelate
S-Monoacetin (gluten free, food additive, also used as gelatinizing agent in explosives and leather tanning)
S-Monocalcium Phosphate
S-Monoglyceride (unmodified)
S-Monoisopropyl Citrate
S-Monopotassium Phosphate
S-Monosaccharides
?-Monosodium Glutamate (see MSG)
S-Monostearates
?-MSG (can be made from seaweed, wheat, or corn; always side with caution)
S-Mung Bean
S-Musk
S-Mustard powder or sauce (verify all ingredients)
S-Myristic Acid
S-Natamycin
?-Natural Flavors (vague, remember wheat is natural)
?-Natural Juices (vague)
S-Natural Smoke Flavor

S-Neotame (gluten free, but toxic)
S-Niacin
S-Niacinamide
N-Nishasta
S-Nitrates
S-Nitric Acid
S-Nitrogen
S-Nitrous Oxide
S-Nori (caution, may contain fillers)
S-Nuts (watch for risk of cross contamination in the roasting process and seasonings)
?-Oat, Oatmeal, Oatrim (see "all grains"; also risk of cross contamination, try to buy from a GF dedicated facility)
S-Oleic Acid
S-Oleoresin
S-Olestra (brand name Olean, gluten free, but a very harmful product found in many potato chips)
S-Oleyl Alcohol/Oil
S-Olive Oil
S-Orange B
S-Orchil
N-Oriental Wheat (triticum turanicum)
N-Oryzanol (usually rice bran oil, corn or barley)
?-Orzenin (see "all grains")
N-Orzo Pasta
S-Oxystearin
S-Ozone

S-Palmitate
S-Palmitic Acid
S-Palm Kernel Oil (gluten free, but coconut oil is more environmentally friendly)
?-Panicin (see "all grains")
S-Pancreatin
S-Pantothenic Acid
S-Papain
S-Paprika
S-Paraffin
N-Pasta (standard is wheat, tons of gluten free varieties available though)
S-Pea - Chick
S-Pea - Cow
S-Pea Flour
S-Peanut (caution with roasted or seasoned)
S-Peanut Flour
S-Peanut Oil
N-Pearl Barley
N-Pearl Rice
S-Peas
S-Pea Starch
S-Pectin
S-Pectinase
S-Pentosanase
S-Peppermint Oil
S-Peppers
S-Pepsin
N-Peptide Bonded Glutamine (usually wheat)

S-Peracetic Acid
N-Persian Wheat (triticum carthlicum)
S-Peru Balsam
N-Perungayam
S-Petrolatum
S-PGPR (Polyglycerol Polyricinoleate)
S-Phenylalanine
S-Phosphate (Calcium)
S-Phosphoric Acid
S-Phosphoric Glycol
S-Phosphorus Oxychloride
S-Pigeon Peas
S-Poi
?-Polenta (corn – see "all grains")
?-Polished Rice (see "all grains")
N-Polish Wheat (triticum polonicum)
S-Polydextrose
S-Polyethylene Glycol
S-Polyglycerol
S-Polyglycerol Polyricinoleate (PGPR)
S-Polysorbates
?-Popcorn (see "all grains")
?-Popcorn Rice (see "all grains")
N-Porter
S-Potassium Acid Tartrate
S-Potassium Benzoate
S-Potassium Bicarbonate
S-Potassium Bisulphite
S-Potassium Carbonate

S-Potassium Carrageenan
S-Potassium Caseinate
S-Potassium Citrate
S-Potassium Fumarate
S-Potassium Furcelleran
S-Potassium Hydroxide
S-Potassium lodate
S-Potassium lodide
S-Potassium Lactate
S-Potassium Matabisulphite
S-Potassium Nitrate
S-Potassium Phosphate
S-Potassium Sorbate
S-Potassium Stearate
S-Potassium Sulphate
S-Potassium Tartrate
S-Potato
?-Potato Chips (look for specific GF products; usually unsafe due to seasonings and processing methods)
S-Potato Flour
S-Potato Starch
N-Poulard Wheat (triticum turgidum)
S-Povidone
?-Powdered Sugar (may contain gluten filler)
?-Pregelatinized Starch (may be from any starch)
N-Pretzels (many GF varieties available)
S-Prinus
S-Pristane
?-Prolamin (vague, see "all grains")

S-Propionic Acid
S-Propolis
S-Propylene Glycol
S-Propylene Glycol Monosterate
S-Propyl Gallate
S-Protease
N-Protein Hydrolysates
S-Psyllium
S-Pullulanase
S-Pyridoxine Hydrochloride
S-Pyrophosphate
S-Quinoa (risk of cross-contamination)
N-Ragi (also called finger or African millet)
S-Raisin Vinegar
S-Rape (see Canola)
S-Recaldent
?-Red Rice (see "all grains")
S-Reduced Iron
S-Rennet
S-Rennet Casein
S-Resinous Glaze
S-Reticulin
S-Riboflavin
?-Rice (see "all grains")
?-Rice Bran
?-Rice Bran Oil
?-Rice Flour
N-Rice Malt (can also contain barley or Koji)
?-Rice Milk

?-Rice Paper
?-Rice Polishings
?-Rice Starch
N-Rice Syrup (barley enzymes)
S-Rice Vinegar (check all ingredients, safe if distilled)
S-Ricinoleic Acid
?-Risotto (Italian rice, see "all grains")
S-Romano Bean (chickpea)
N-Roquefort Cheese (listed as safe on most lists but usually contains trace amounts of gluten)
S-Rosematta
S-Rosin
?-Rough Rice (see "all grains")
N-Roux (thickener, usually wheat flour)
S-Royal Jelly
N-Rusk
N-Rye
S-Saccharin
S-Safflower Oil (many Celiacs have reactions)
S-Saffron
S-Sago
S-Sago Flour or Starch
S-Sago Palm
S-Saifun (bean threads)
S-Salba
S-Salt
S-Saponin
?-Sausage (check for fillers)
?-Seasonings (caution with vague terms)

S-Seaweed (plain dry versions are safe and very good for you; caution with snack versions that have added flavors like soy & teriyaki, which are unsafe)
N-Secalin
N-Seitan
N-Semolina
N-Semolina Triticum
S-Sesame
S-Sesame Butter (if pure)
S-Shea
S-Sherry Vinegar
N-Shortening (can contain vitamin E from wheat germ)
N-Shot Wheat (triticum aestivum)
N-Shoyu
S-Silicon Dioxide
N-Sirimi (binder: usually wheat or cornstarch)
N-Small Spelt
S-Soba (verify it is 100% buckwheat; also high risk of cross contamination)
S-Sodium Acetate
S-Sodium Acid Pyrophosphate
S-Sodium Alginate
S-Sodium Ascorbate
S-Sodium Benzoate
?-Sodium Caseinate (contains MSG)
S-Sodium Citrate
S-Sodium Erythrobate
S-Sodium Hexametaphosphate
S-Sodium Lactate

S-Sodium Lauryl Sulfate (gluten free, but harmful product found in synthetic soap, shampoo, detergents – try to replace with phosphate free, natural products)
S-Sodium Metabisulphite
S-Sodium Nitrate
S-Sodium Phosphate
S-Sodium Polyphosphate
S-Sodium Silaco Aluminate
?-Sodium Starch Glycolate (may be from any starch)
S-Sodium Stearoyl Lactylate
S-Sodium Sulphite
S-Sodium Stannate
S-Sodium Tripolyphosphate
N-Soft Wheat
S-Sorbic Acid
S-Sorbitan Monostearate
S-Sorbitan Trioleate
S-Sorbitan Tristearate
S-Sorbitol-Mannitol (can cause IBS symptoms)
?-Sorghum (see "all grains")
?-Sorgum (see "all grains")
S-Soy (gluten free but many Celiacs sensitive to all soy; standard soy sauce unsafe – gluten added)
S-Soya Flour
S-Soya Starch
S-Soybean
S-Soy Lecithin

S-Soy Milk (check for added flavors or malt)
S-Soy Protein
S-Soy Protein Isolate
N-Soy Sauce
N-Spelt (triticum spelta)
S-Sphingolipids Soba (safe if it is 100% buckwheat)
?-Spices (verify for fillers)
?-Spirits (see alcohol)
N-Sprouted Wheat or Barley
?-Stabilizers (verify source)
?-Starch (can be made from many sources)
N-Stativa
S-Stearamide
S-Stearamine
S-Stearates
S-Stearic Acid
S-Stearyl Citrate
N-Stearyldimoniumhydroxypropyl Hydrolyzed Wheat Protein
S-Stearyl Lactate
S-Stevia
N-Stock Cubes
N-Strong Flour
N-Stout
S-Streptococcus Thermophilus
S-Subflower Seed
S-Succinic Anhydride
?-Succotash (beans & corn: see "all grains"/corn)

S-Sucralose
S-Sucrose
S-Suet, raw fat safe (dried packet suet unsafe)
S-Sugar (pure form safe, caution with powdered sugar)
S-Sulfites
S-Sulfosuccinate
S-Sulfur Dioxide
S-Sulphuric Acid
S-Sulphurous Acid
S-Sunflower oil or seed
N-Surimi
S-Sweet Chestnut Flour
S-Sweet Potato
?-Sweet Rice Flour (see "all grains")
S-Tagatose
S-Tahini (100% pure sesame)
S-Tallow
N-Tamari
S-Tamarind
S-Tannic Acid
S-Tapioca
S-Tapioca Flour
S-Tapioca Starch
S-Tara Gum
S-Taro
S-Tarro
S-Tarrow Root
S-Tartaric Acid
S-Tartrazine (gluten free, but harmful to health)

S-TBHQ - tertiary butylhydroquinone (gluten free preservative, but shown to be toxic in studies)
S-Tea (check for added ingredients, I recommend whole tea leaves; caution with Genmaicha which may be made with barley instead of rice)
S-Tea Tree Oil
S-Teff (cross contamination risk)
?-Tempeh (often contains soy sauce)
S-Tepary Bean
N-Teriyaki Sauce
?-Texmati Rice (see "all grains")
?-Textured Vegetable Protein (wheat or soy)
S-Thaumatin
S-Thiamine Hydrochloride
S-Thiamine Mononitrate
N-Timopheevi Wheat (triticum timopheevii)
S-Titanium Dioxide
S-Tocopherols
S-Tofu (check for added ingredients)
S-Tolu Balsam
N-Tortillas
S-Torula Yeast
N-Tostada
S-Tragacanth
S-Tragacanth Gum
S-Triacetin
S-Tributyrin
S-Tricalcium Phosphate

S-Triethyl Citrate
N-Triticale X Triticosecale
N-Triticum Vulgare (wheat) Germ Extract or Oil
S-Trypsin
S-Turmeric
?-TVP (can be wheat or soy)
S-Tyrosine
N-Udon (usually wheat, sometimes corn)
N-Unbleached Flour
S-Urad/Urid Beans
S-Urad/Urid Dal (peas) Vegetables
S-Urad/Urid flour
S-Urd
?-Valencia Rice (see "all grains")
S-Vanilla Extract (pure vanilla)
S-Vanilla Flavoring (verify it is pure vanilla)
S-Vanillin
N-Vavilovi Wheat (triticum aestivum)
?-Vegetable Broth (vague)
?-Vegetable Gum (verify grains)
?-Vegetable Protein
N-Vegetable shortening
?-Vegetable Starch (verify contents)
?-Vinegar (apple cider, wine, and balsamic are usually safe; see vinegar in the "hidden sources" chapter)
N-Vital Wheat Gluten
N-Vulgar
?-Waxy Maize (see "all grains")
?-Wehani Rice (see "all grains")

N-Wheat, abyssinian hard triticum durum
N-Wheat Amino Acids
N-Wheat Bran
N-Wheat Bran Extract
N-Wheat Bulgur
N-Wheat Durum Triticum
N-Wheat Germ
?-Wheat Germamidopropyldimonium Hydroxypropyl (processing method might eliminate gluten content)
N-Wheat Germ Glycerides
N-Wheat Germ Oil
S-Wheatgrass (grass portion is safe, the seeds are not; if cutting to juice, cut 1cm away from seed)
N-Wheat Nuts
N-Wheat Protein
N-Wheat Triticum Aestivum
N-Wheat Triticum Monococcum
S-Whey (pure whey safe; modified versions may contain trace amounts of gluten; for supplement shake powders read the label carefully)
S-Whey Protein Concentrate
S-Whey Protein Isolate
N-White Grain Vinegar
N-Whole-Meal Flour
N-Whole Wheat Berries
N-Whole Wheat Flour
N-Wild Einkorn (triticum boeotictim)
N-Wild Emmer (triticum dicoccoides)

?-Wild Rice (see "all grains")
S-Wine -standard wine* is safe; wine coolers not safe (*note: some winemakers use fining agents that contain gluten, plus there are manufacturers of the oak wine barrels themselves that use flour paste when sealing the oak slabs-which I have personally watched by a manufacturer in France. You may consider verifying with your favorite vintners).
N-Wine coolers
S-Wine Vinegar (safe, see vinegar)
S-Wood Smoke
N-Worcestershire (usually contains barley)
S-Xanthophyll
?-Xanthum Gum (can be made from wheat, soy, corn, or dairy)
S-Xylanase
S-Xylitol
S-Yam
S-Yam Flour
?-Yeast (Autolyzed, Baker's, Nutritional, Torula safe; Brewer's not safe. often grown or dried on wheat flour, side with caution, buy specially marked GF versions)
S-Yogurt (caution with added flavors, fruit, toppings; added muesli or granola unsafe)
?-Zein (see "all grains")
S-Zinc Oxide
S-Zinc Sulfate

+++++

THE LAW – HOW "LEGAL AMOUNTS" ARE KILLING YOU FASTER

A few days before I went to print with this book, an esteemed doctor who is one of the most noted on Celiac Disease released a statement saying he felt that not lowering legally accepted amounts of gluten would make life easier for everyone, both the patient (who wouldn't have to be on such high alert) and manufacturers (who wouldn't have to worry about small variances). He went on to say that the studies showing reactions to "small amounts" of gluten should not be paid attention to because they weren't across the board. I wonder how he would feel if his child was in that "small number" and I wonder if he is aware that children with Celiac Disease have a threefold higher risk of long-term mortality[4,] and adults at 39%[1].

People with gluten sensitivity resulting in inflammation have over 70% risk to higher mortality rates[1]. ...70% and they're not even officially diagnosed allergic.

I can't express how disappointed I was to hear him talk, and my reasons follow in this section.

Other than acknowledging my discontent, I have not changed one word from my original position on ppm's but wanted to mention it in case you came across it too and it created confusion.

I will be shunned by all the Celiac Associations over this article, but since when was progress ever made by following the pack?

I am more than happy to stand out on the ledge by myself and loudly disagree with what the government agencies are doing and make clear that I disagree with Celiac Associations that are all just endorsing the "legal" amounts instead of questioning something that is really a health hazard for their members.

What amount of gluten is safe for a Celiac? Legally in most countries it is presently 10-20ppm. In Australia it used to be 20ppm, legal amount is now 5, and for a product to be labeled GF it must be less than 3. The Codex standard in the UK was 200ppm in 1981, changed to 20ppm in 2008. Finland is still at 100ppm. In America the FDA is proposing 20ppm, Canada is introducing new laws in 2012 and so it goes from country to country, ranging from 3 to 500ppm.

They keep modifying to lower & lower quantities... meanwhile what about the people who have been digesting the old "legal" amounts all these years? Good question, to which there is no answer – they are clearly on their own, destined to become the statistics of the coming decades.

Here are my issues with all these "legal amounts" of gluten (studies at end of book if you are interested):

There has been no extensive long-term research done on Celiac Disease because most research is funded by pharmaceutical companies. These companies have no interest in funding research for a condition that requires only a change in diet and that they can't sell any drugs to, not to mention limits their cu$tomer base to 1% of the population. I am not convinced of data that is released when the topic hasn't been exhaustively and objectively studied with double-blind tests and end outcome not pre-determined by the sponsors of the study.

Of the studies that have been done, look at the wording closely and you will see that there are always words like "preliminary", "inconclusive", and other words that offer escape hatches. If the results are inconclusive, why use those numbers to instate laws? Why not wait until we know what we are talking about conclusively and without a doubt?

The agencies that set the laws, such as the FDA and their counterparts worldwide, are under major pressure from manufacturers to set the legal amounts to high levels; they do this so that it won't require the manufacturers to go the expensive route of creating entirely GF lines in their plants. Canada's new laws for 2012 state that consideration of any and all cross-contamination is omitted - which means regardless of the 20ppm legal limit (which is already questionable), using the cross-contamination loophole, a product can contain ANY amount of gluten and still be labeled GF legally. Wow. A loophole the size of Texas on a subject that shuts down the consumer's intestines. *Great job Canada.* I seem to be the only person in the country who read the actual content of the law while everyone else is applauding the headline.

These government agencies are the same ones that told us smoking was safe for 60 years, are now allowing lethally harmful laws for GMO's to go into effect, said arsenic based pesticides were safe for 40 years, allowed use of DDT since the 50's, allow Atrazine to still be legal in the Americas today (yet illegal in its country of origin and banned in Europe), legalize and even enforce administration of highly harmful vaccines that have killed and irreversibly damaged hundreds of thousands of people – these are all big deals affecting 100% of the population and they knew/know what they are doing. Do you trust these very same agencies with the safety limits they set on gluten when it is relatively minor, affecting a smaller percentage of the population, and they have no idea what they are doing... and I might add, with no way to immediately measure the harm done to the body with these "safe trace amounts of contamination"??? It's not like gluten contamination is causing anaphylactic shocks and would raise immediate flags; it's a slow silent killer that eats away at a person's health and impossible to measure in the short term for most.

We know that the smallest amount of just one contamination can create harmful antibodies that remain in a Celiac for up to 6 months – how could small constant trace amounts be safe? Is the cumulative effect even being considered?

Every country and university on earth has conflicting amounts they deem as safe, all studies outright admit their conclusions as inconclusive and premature, all these studies show people were forced to drop out of the study midway due to harmful complications while they were testing the "trace amounts" – yet we are accepting 20ppm as safe? And the "dropouts" are omitted from the final conclusions because they weren't in the study beginning to end. *Gotta love that. Unreal.*

If we take a clear large pitcher of water and put one tiny drop of red ink into it, it changes the chemical make-up of the water. Wouldn't common sense conclude that ANY amount of gluten is unsafe?

Now here's what to watch out for in coming years: now that there are several million potential lifetime cu$tomer$, the lifelong magic pills will hit the shelves and prescription pads, as they have already begun to do. Do not allow yourself to become a victim by trusting your doctor and government – we only need to look at the corruption of psychotropic drugs to know that we need to use our own judgment and do our own research.

As a Celiac myself, **I refuse to play *Gluten Roulette* with my health** while the medical world keeps changing its findings and the pharma world slowly places its commercial arm on the matter.

I don't believe in telling people what to do, but I strongly believe in informed choices. I think people should be aware of what is really happening with studies and all the discrepancies in them and we should have a right to know whether food that is marked as GF is truly 100% GF or if there may be trace amounts – and allow each individual to decide for themselves whether they will consume that product or not.

I am against government setting a legal limit that is unconfirmed without any conclusive & extensive long term studies and allowing companies to use the gluten free labels under ambiguous numbers. Just mark 20ppm on the box and specify if the facility is 100% dedicated GF and let me decide if I will risk it or not.

Informed choices. Transparency. Freedom to choose. These are what I feel are every person's right.

[studies and additional information added to the "references section" at the end of this book]

YOU CAN BE SUPER HEALTHY!

THE MOST IMPORTANT HEALTH FACTOR THAT IS ALWAYS IGNORED

Generally what happens when you are diagnosed with gluten sensitivity or Celiac Disease is that you are told there is no cure and that you must avoid gluten. And the conversation ends there... *if you're lucky.* If you're not lucky you will be pointed to a flawed outdated list and continue to feel sick, which your doctor will say is "normal". FYI docs, "sick" is not "normal"; health is.

The other tragedy that happens (I know the intentions are good all the way around, don't send me hate mail for saying this) but you might be directed to a nutritionist who has zero experience with gluten free diets and they will be looking things up in the same flawed lists everyone else has. *"Blind leading the blind".*

Here is the element everyone is ignoring: your system has sustained severe damage and needs help to heal. You need to be eating and drinking foods to boost your immune system back up so that your body can start to fight off its attackers – a.k.a. inflammation, antibodies, and who knows what else!

Re-building the immune system must be priority 1.

RECOVERY STRATEGY

This section is next to impossible to write because every individual is at a different stage of damage. Every individual was also at a different level of health before being diagnosed.

First and foremost get thorough blood work done and see where there are deficiencies. If you have intestinal damage like I did, your body won't be doing a good job of absorbing vitamins via pills. Find lozenge or liquid forms so that you can melt them under your tongue – that goes right into your bloodstream. Vitamin B_{12}, iron, and many of the vitamins and minerals that commonly will show up as deficiencies are available in various forms. Work closely with your doctor on this and ask for a copy of all blood test results.

Next, consider what your body has been through and give it a much deserved rest. Your digestive system probably needs a vacation and your intestinal tract probably needs repair. Find a naturopath in your area and have them help you through a nutritionally strong juice fast. Don't do this on your own unless you are qualified, but a nutritionally complete and dense juice diet is the best way to both heal and strengthen at the same time.

The key to fast recovery and then maintenance is concentrated greens. Green juices, smoothies, soups, salads. Dark leafy (organic) greens are really powerful.

Again working with someone qualified, evaluate your diet. Just cutting out gluten is not enough, you need to do damage control. You want to eliminate everything that will stress or overwork your body (even if only for a while).

Obviously I never suggest a bad diet, so I am not suggesting you eat well for a month and then return to junk food – but I am realistic and know that chances are the majority of you reading this don't have "excellent" food habits and the majority of you are not going to give up foods you know aren't necessarily great. At least do it for a few months while your body recovers. You owe yourself that much. And if you return to eating not-so-great food, be conscious of it and try to 1) not do that every day 2) at least compensate by adding lots of fruits and vegetables and powerful dishes to help balance things out.

Not to be self-promoting here, but my "NakedFood" book is specifically designed to boost your immune system. Every recipe from fun dips to luscious desserts is engineered to power you up. So you don't need to completely adopt my diet, but do add my dishes to your overall diet here and there and I promise it will help.

Common sense is your best friend right now. Your body has been under attack, do what you can to help it heal and re-build. Dark greens are your best friend! Let me help you get started…

AMAZING HEALING DRINKS

1) ALOE VERA JUICE

It doesn't just heal burns, when taken orally it heals internally as well. You don't want to buy the "gel", you want to buy the "juice". Certified organic aloe vera juice. You want to drink at least 2 ounces of it every day, particularly in the initial recovery stage.

Word of warning, it tastes quite bitter – but the good news is that it is very easy to cover up that taste.

Get out your martini shaker (I used to laugh doing that at 7am) and just shake up the aloe juice with a juice that has a very strong flavor so that it will cover up the bitterness.

My choices were cranberry or pomegranate – both of which have excellent properties of their own. (needless to say, not the sugar loaded cocktail juices but the pure organic unsweetened juices, add organic maple syrup or raw honey if you need to sweeten)

Declare cocktail hour every day, make it enjoyable, and the healing will take place that much faster. I used to drink them from a martini glass!

2) SPIRULINA

A great source for the elusive B_{12} (mineral rich earth is still the best source for B_{12}, though next to impossible to find, making Spirulina the next best source due to availability), good source of vitamins B_1, B_2, B_3, B_6, C, D, E, K, folic acid, pantothenic acid, biotin, inositol, calcium, magnesium, potassium, phosphorus (is in every cell throughout the body and works with calcium to maintain bone density), chromium, selenium, and great source for iron (10x higher than normal foods).

The phycocyanin (blue pigment) in spirulina combines with iron and other minerals making them more bio-available (2x more than meats and vegetables).

10g of spirulina provides 23,000 I.U. of beta carotene which the body converts to Vitamin A (which is a particularly important vitamin for people with autoimmune disorders like Celiac because it helps heal the intestinal tract); and unlike taking Vitamin A supplements (fat soluble, too much can be toxic), when it is your body doing the converting, it automatically stops at the right amount. *Such a miraculous thing the body is, in its natural form.* Beta carotene is a powerful antioxidant that fights free radicals and also reduces the body's risks to several types of cancer including colon and gastrointestinal tract.

Spirulina is a complete protein that delivers all essential amino acids in a highly absorbable form.

As well as zeaxanthin and lutein which are important for vision – blindness is actually becoming a bigger and bigger issue.

Low in sodium making this superfood appropriate for salt-restricted diets (90mg per 10g) and it contains no bad cholesterol.

Spirulina strengthens the immune system while simultaneously helping the body detoxify.

RECIPE FOR MY "POWER BLUE TONIC"
IN BLENDER:
1 cup blueberries (fresh or frozen)
1 heaping tbsp spirulina
1 tsp raw cacao (antioxidants and delicious!)
1 cup coconut water (or plain water, but coconut water add electrolytes)
1 tbsp blackstrap molasses (adds iron)
1 tsp wheat grass powder (certified GF)
1-2 oz aloe vera juice (healing properties)
7-8 walnuts (omega-3's)
3-5 Brazil nuts (organic, high in selenium)
3-4 Medjool dates (optional, this adds sweetness, but also highly usable raw energy)

Now THAT'S what I call a power drink!

3) **MINT**

...you'll be pleasantly surprised...

• excellent for anyone with digestive disorders, stomach aches

• has a calming effect, used to help with headaches, depression, and insomnia

• contains menthol, thymol, carvacrol – all fight flatulence

• increases perspiration, thereby decreasing fever

• protects the liver and helps it function more efficiently

• reduces pain for those with gallstones or kidney stones

• antifungal properties are fantastic to help relieve issues in the respiratory tract and asthma issues

• helps with diarrhea and IBS discomfort

• improves blood circulation

• contains perillyl alcohol, an anti-cancer property

• decreases altitude sickness (hikers/climbers, start having infusions from 3-4 days ahead)

• its antioxidants are said to prevent cataracts (though you would need to consume several cups every day to intake enough for this)

• last but not least, it even freshens the breath, so enjoy your minty drinks and make sure you kiss a loved one!

RECIPE FOR "MOJITO WITH A TWIST"

--Crush a handful of mint (mortar & pestle are best, but improvise if you don't have them, you can use a wooden spoon or just chop & smash), along with a small piece of fresh ginger and the juice of ½ a lime

(you can add maple syrup if you'd like some sweetness, do avoid toxic white sugar as most mojito recipes call for)

--Put the mixture in a tall glass, add ice & water, and think of something wonderful to toast to!

Of course you read the long list of benefits from the mint, but don't underestimate the anti-inflammatory strength of the fresh ginger as well. It seems like a simple drink, but it is seriously powerful.

REFERENCES

[1]JAMA, Sept 16, 2009, Vol 302, No.11

[2]Dig Dis Sci (2010) 55:1026-1031

[3]Eur J of Endocrinology (2002) 146 479-483

[4]Am J Gastroenterol 2007;102:864-870

[5]Mehr S, Kakakios A, et al. Food Protein Induced Enterocolitis Syndrome: 16 year experience. Pediatrics 2009; 123(3):e459-3464.

[6]Mehr S, Kakakios A, et al. Rice: a common and severe cause of food protein induced enterocolitis syndrome. Arch Dis Child 2009;94(3):220-3.

[7]"Maize prolamines had low but definite activity even though maize is reported to be harmless" Gut, 1983,24,825-830

[8]"The allergens in rice, corn, millet, and buckwheat should be better studied before they can be recommended as alternatives for cereal allergic children." Clin Exp Allergy 1995 Nov;25(11):1100-7.

[9]"High titres were also found...tested against wheat glutenins, albumins, and globulins, as well as against barley, oats, and maize prolamines" J Pediatr Gastroenterol Nutr. 1987 May Jun;6(3):346-50.

[10]University of Chicago Celiac Research

ADDITIONAL INFORMATION FROM THE "THE LAW" SECTION REGARDING PPM

>> I have spent endless hours analyzing studies from around the world and have yet to find one, *just one*, which conclusively states a certain amount of gluten was absolutely safe long term and that none of the patients in their study had any adverse reactions. Some, like the first study I have listed below, outright state a safe number cannot be determined yet. Let's look at just a few studies and my comments follow the ">>" marks.

--Curr Opin Clin Nutr Metab Care. 2008 May;11(3):329-33.

--Issues related to gluten-free diet in coeliac disease.

--Troncone R, Auricchio R, Granata V.

--Department of Pediatrics and European Laboratory for the Investigation of Food-Induced Diseases, University Federico II, Naples, Italy.

"RECENT FINDINGS: Gluten-free diet is generally admitted as effective therapy in symptomatic patients, but a life-long dietary treatment in some challenging cases such as 'silent' and 'latent' patients is under discussion. Tolerance to gluten may be acquired later

in life, but, as latency may be transient, a strict follow-up is necessary in these patients. The composition of gluten-free diet needs a better definition; latest evidence demonstrates that oats are tolerated by most patients with coeliac disease. Finally, the amount of gluten permitted in gluten-free products is still a matter of debate; significant progress has been made in the sensitivity of techniques for gluten detection, but the daily amount of gluten that can be safely consumed is not yet defined."

>> I can't help but wonder, if there WAS any safe amount, wouldn't they have found it while experimenting?

--Aliment Pharmacol Ther. 2008 Jun 1;27(11):1044-52. Epub 2008 Feb 29.

--Systematic review: tolerable amount of gluten for people with coeliac disease.

--Akobeng AK, Thomas AG.

--Department of Paediatric Gastroenterology, Booth Hall Children's Hospital, Central Manchester and Manchester Children's University Hospitals, Manchester, UK.

"RESULTS: Thirteen studies (three randomized controlled, one cohort, two crossover, and seven cross-

sectional) met the inclusion criteria. The daily amount of tolerable gluten varied widely between studies. Whilst some patients tolerated an average of 34-36 mg of gluten per day, other patients who consumed about 10 mg of gluten per day developed mucosal abnormalities. The effect of the consumption of 'gluten-free' products with different degrees of gluten contamination was also inconsistent.

>> note: 10mg is set as the legal amount in many countries, and this study clearly showed: "*...developed mucosal abnormalities*".

CONCLUSIONS: The amount of tolerable gluten varies among people with coeliac disease. Although there is no evidence to suggest a single definitive threshold, a daily gluten intake of <10 mg is unlikely to cause significant histological abnormalities."

>>> "unlikely" means it will not affect everyone the same way and the fact is they don't even know what the long term effects are because studies don't last more than a few weeks. ...back to the Celiac Roulette game I mentioned... They are handling gluten the way they handle vaccines: if it kills or paralyzes only a small % of people, then it's not a significant enough risk for them to stop it.

--American Journal of Clinical Nutrition, Vol. 85, No. 1, 160-166, January 2007

--A prospective, double-blind, placebo-controlled trial to establish a safe gluten threshold for patients with celiac disease [1,2,3]

-- Carlo Catassi, et al.

--[2] Supported in part by the Italian Celiac Society. Purified gluten was kindly supplied by Bruno Jarry while working for the Tate & Lyle Group (United Kingdom).

--[3] Reprints not available. Address correspondence to A Fasano, Mucosal Biology Research Center, University of Maryland School of Medicine, 20 Penn Street, Room 345, Baltimore, MD 21201

THEIR CONCLUSION is clearly saying they do not know if ANY amount of gluten is safe for a Celiac: *"In conclusion, this study confirmed that an abnormal small-bowel morphology persisted in a significant proportion of CD patients being treated with a GFD, most likely because of the persistent ingestion of trace amounts of gluten. The protracted intake of 50 mg gluten/d produced significant damage in the architecture of the small intestine in patients being treated for CD. However, the sensitivity to trace intakes of gluten showed large interpatient variability, a feature that should be accounted for in the implementation of a safe gluten threshold. These findings should be confirmed by further studies in larger numbers of CD patients. Finally, the relation between the intestinal damage induced by trace intakes of gluten and* <u>*the long-term complications of CD remains to be elucidated*</u>*."*

>> An interesting thing to note about this study - several people had to be dropped every step of the way during the study due to intolerable pain or apparent damage being caused – I will use direct quotes from the study:

"4 of 49 subjects had to be excluded from the protocol because severe enteropathy"

"Furthermore, one patient challenged with 10 mg gluten/d experienced clinical symptoms after a few weeks, whereas none of the 13 subjects receiving 50 mg gluten/d had clinical evidence of relapse."

"One patient (challenged with 10 mg gluten) developed a clinical relapse."

"7 of the 49 patients had to be excluded because of abnormal small-intestinal histology, development of thyroid carcinoma, or gastric polyposis confirmed by gastroduodenoscopy or because the subject refused randomization."

"Three other cases did not complete the microchallenge because of change of residence (1 challenged with 50 mg), poor adherence to the protocol (1 challenged with 10 mg), or development of symptoms (1 challenged with 10 mg)"

"One patient challenged with 10 mg gluten/d showed typical signs of relapse (vomiting, diarrhea, and abdominal distension) after 6–8 wk of microchallenge but refused to repeat the t_1 *evaluation."*

>> If such a small study caused havoc for so many of the participants, would that not indicate that no amount of gluten should be concluded as safe, as indeed their final conclusion says: "*CD remains to be elucidated*".

--Aliment Pharmacol Ther. 2004 Jun 15;19(12):1277-83.

--The safe threshold for gluten contamination in gluten-free products. Can trace amounts be accepted in the treatment of coeliac disease?

--Collin P, Thorell L, Kaukinen K, Mäki M.

--Department of Medicine, Tampere University Hospital, and Medical School, University of Tampere, Tampere, Finland.

"RESULTS: A number of both naturally gluten-free (13 of 59) and wheat starch-based gluten-free (11 of 24) products contained gluten from 20 to 200 ppm (=mg/kg). The median daily flour consumption was 80 g (range: 10-300). Within these limits, the long-term mucosal recovery was good."

>> Finland has based its legal amount at 100ppm based on a study that says "long-term mucosal recovery was good"

a) They are clearly stating there was damage incurred when talking about recovery time; so as long as recovery is possible then it's ok to knowingly incur damage?

b) This was based on how many contaminations within their study? Obviously not years of constant amounts... there is a scary follow-up report that will appear in the short years ahead following this study.

>> The final fact is that the only conclusive statement that can be made on the issue of safe amounts of gluten is that there is no way to make a conclusive statement regarding any level higher than zero.

To book Jaqui for a speaking engagement please email: info [at] JaquiKarr.com

Library and Archives Canada

Author: Karr, Jaqui

Title: “What Is Gluten and What Is Gluten In”

ISBN: 978-0-9869039-4-6

Made in the USA
Lexington, KY
06 June 2012